新冠肺炎药物
指导手册
（中英对照版）

主　编　杨宝峰

副主编　郭　姣　张　莹　梁海海　张　勇

编　委（按姓氏笔画排序）

卞　宇　白云龙　刘　鑫　许超千

孙　宁　杜伟杰　杨　磊　杨宝峰

肖　雪　张　洋　张　勇　张　莹

陈　畅　单宏丽　赵一秀　宣立娜

郭　姣　梁海海　蔡本志　潘振伟

人民卫生出版社

图书在版编目（CIP）数据

新冠肺炎药物指导手册：中英对照版 / 杨宝峰主编
. —北京：人民卫生出版社，2020.3
ISBN 978-7-117-29872-8

Ⅰ.①新… Ⅱ.①杨… Ⅲ.①日冕形病毒 — 病毒病 —
肺炎 — 药物 — 临床应用 — 手册 — 汉、英 Ⅳ.①R974-62

中国版本图书馆 CIP 数据核字（2020）第 036581 号

人卫智网	**www.ipmph.com**	医学教育、学术、考试、健康，
		购书智慧智能综合服务平台
人卫官网	**www.pmph.com**	人卫官方资讯发布平台

新冠肺炎药物指导手册
（中英对照版）

主　　编：杨宝峰
出版发行：人民卫生出版社（中继线 010-59780011）
地　　址：北京市朝阳区潘家园南里 19 号
邮　　编：100021
E - mail：pmph @ pmph.com
购书热线：010-59787592　010-59787584　010-65264830
印　　刷：三河市潮河印业有限公司
经　　销：新华书店
开　　本：889×1194　1/32　印张：7.5
字　　数：181 千字
版　　次：2020 年 3 月第 1 版　2020 年 3 月第 1 版第 1 次印刷
标准书号：ISBN 978-7-117-29872-8
定　　价：36.00 元
打击盗版举报电话：010-59787491　E-mail：WQ @ pmph.com
质量问题联系电话：010-59787234　E-mail：zhiliang @ pmph.com

Guide Manual on Pharmacological Management of Coronavirus Disease 2019 (COVID-19)

Chief Editor Yang Baofeng

Vice Chief Editor Guo Jiao Zhang Ying
Liang Haihai Zhang Yong

Contributors

Bian Yu	Bai Yunlong	Liu Xin	Xu Chaoqian
Sun Ning	Du Weijie	Yang Lei	Yang Baofeng
Xiao Xue	Zhang Yang	Zhang Yong	Zhang Ying
Chen Chang	Shan Hongli	Zhao Yixiu	Xuan Lina
Guo Jiao	Liang Haihai	Cai Benzhi	Pan Zhenwei

前　言

　　自 2019 年底,以湖北武汉为中心的新型冠状病毒肺炎(新冠肺炎)疫情在我国各地蔓延,牵动亿万民众之心,造成严重的社会危害。党中央、国务院对此次疫情高度重视,习近平总书记多次作出重要指示,强调要把人民群众生命安全和身体健康放在第一位,尽最大努力、采取更科学周密的措施遏制疫情扩散蔓延态势,坚决打赢疫情防控阻击战。为认真贯彻习近平总书记关于新冠肺炎疫情的重要讲话和重要指示精神,落实国家新冠肺炎疫情联防联控要求,充分发挥科技在抗疫治疗中的作用,以钟南山院士为首的广大医务人员和科研工作者争相投入这场没有硝烟的战斗。

　　国家卫生健康委员会、国家中医药管理局陆续发布了七版《新型冠状病毒肺炎诊疗方案(试行)》,对新冠肺炎的病原学特点、流行病学特点、临床特点、诊断标准及治疗等进行了详细阐述,但目前尚无特效的治疗药物。抗病毒药物作为新冠肺炎一般治疗的常用药物,其存在各自使用的禁忌、相互作用及不良反应等,临床使用过程中应因人制宜、合理使用。糖皮质激素具有强大的抗炎作用,但使用不当会产生严重的副作用。新冠肺炎典型的病理改变为支气管腔内大量黏液及黏液栓的积聚,故本手册编入部分祛痰药。作为中华文明瑰宝,中医药强调"扶正与祛邪"结合,着力于病原体进入人体后邪气与正气斗争所表现的证候而辨证论治,在改善临床症状、减少并发症、提高生活质量等方面具有独到优势。老药新用、中西结合、各有侧重、优势互补,成为治疗新冠肺炎的有效策略。

基于此,编者依据人民卫生出版社《药理学》(第9版)(杨宝峰、陈建国主编)、《新型冠状病毒肺炎诊疗方案(试行第七版)》,参考多部药学专著及临床多中心观察药物进展、国家卫生健康委员会有关通知,结合新冠肺炎的疾病特点,从药物的作用机制、不良反应、配伍禁忌和临床合理用药出发,编制本手册。本手册编入的抗病毒类化学药物、中药及方剂,部分药物尚缺乏对新型冠状病毒肺炎疗效的循证医学证据,仅供临床医护人员及药师等相关人员参考。

限于编者的学识和水平,且时间仓促,本手册不足之处在所难免,请各位读者谅解,并恳请大家批评指正。

杨宝峰

2020年3月3日

Preface

Since the end of 2019, the epidemic of Coronavirus Disease 2019 (COVID-19) centered in Wuhan, Hubei Province, has spread all over China due to the super human-to-human transmission of the virus, which affects the health status and even lives of thousands of people and causes serious public health problems and social/economic burdens.

The Central Committee of Communist Party of China and the State Council attach great importance to the epidemic and have promptly implemented a series of emergent health measures. Upon outbreak of the epidemic in Wuhan and its rapid spreading nationwide which once made the nation entirely caught off guard, Chinese President Xi Jinping has responded immediately to the unanticipated event, formulating strategic deployments for the prevention and control of the epidemic and launching national campaign against the virus. He put particular stress on that governments at all levels and health-related organizations must overwhelmingly place the safety of people's lives and health in the first place and make the best efforts by prioritizing and implementing all necessary measures with the highest scientific and technological standards to terminate spread of COVID-19 until a final win of the battle. The supreme leader's wise decision and firm determination immediately mobilized and motivated the whole nation to take serious and later confirmed to be effective actions consciously and confidently. The medical staffs and researchers led by Dr. Zhong Nanshan (medical doctor, professor and scientist, academician) stand in the front line of the batter fields and self-sacrifice to save and cherish the lives of others, with their full morality and virtue as well as their professional knowledge and skills. We could now declare with great pride that we won the battle and the Chinese model of combating COVID-19 created a miracle and set a benchmark in medicine and in human history ! Yet, while COVID-19 is now well under control within China, the epidemic has become pandemic across more than 130 countries of all continents in this globe. Thus, human battle against COVID-19 is far from over. Nonetheless, a critical situation we human beings are facing is the overall lack of practical experience and guidelines in the management of patients who carry COVID-19.

National Health Commission of the People's Republic of China has issued seven editions of *Guidelines for the Diagnosis and Treatment of COVID-19* (Tentative 7th Edition) , elaborating the etiology, epidemiological characteristics, clinical characteristics, diagnostic criteria, clinical manifestations and treatment of COVID-19. Unfortunately, at present there have not been any proven effective and safe anti-coronavirus drugs for clinical applications. Even though, antiviral and anti-inflammatory agents are frequently used as "better-than-nothing" treatment of COVID-19 in China. However, while these drugs have demonstrated varying degrees of effectiveness against COVID-19, they in general come with various contraindications, unwanted drug interactions and adverse reactions, in addition to their uncertain efficacy. For example, glucocorticoids have strong anti-inflammatory effects, but they can cause serious side effects if used improperly. Clearly, there is an urgent need to clarify and standardize the clinical applications of these drugs for COVID-19.

The most noticeable and typical pathological outcome of COVID-19 is an accumulation of a large volume of mucus and mucus suppository in the bronchial lumen, which is presumably caused by inflammation storm. The content on segmental expectorants is therefore covered in this manual. On the other hand, traditional Chinese medicine (TCM) emphasizes the concept of "FUZHENGQUXIE (invigorate the body defense and resistance systems and dispel pathogenic factors)" in combating diseases and the approach of symptom-based therapy focusing on suppressing evil Qi (energy) and mobilizing healthy Qi. During the campaign against COVID-19, TCM has been employed alone or in combination with modern western medicine. In either way, TCM has demonstrated its appealing successfulness and unique advantages in improving clinical symptoms of COVID-19 and eliminating the virus from body, particularly in blocking the transition or degeneration of mild patients to critical ones and in reversing the critical patients as well by reducing complications and improving quality of life. Such advantages have also been evidenced in the patients of Italian population who received TCM treatment. It is therefore not exaggerated to state that the strategy of old drugs—new uses and combination of TCM and western medicine with mutual complementing advantages appears to be superior for the treatment of COVID-19. Hence, TCM is also included in this manual.

In preparing this book, the editorial board members followed the basic principles of *Pharmacology* (9th Edition), People's Medical Publishing House (Edited by Yang Baofeng and Chen Jianguo) and *Guidelines for the Diagnosis and Treatment of COVID-19* (Tentative 7th Edition), consulted several pharmaceutics monographs and incorporated the most updated knowledge about the COVID-19 from clinical practice and trials. This book aims to elaborate the pharmacological action, adverse reactions, incompatibility and clinical rational use of drugs and provide a basic reference guide for the pharmacological management of COVID-19. Overall, this manual covers the contents on antiviral drugs, traditional Chinese medicine and prescriptions. It must be noted that this manual is prepared as a reference guide for clinical medical staffs, pharmacists and other health-related personnel in fighting COVID-19 and it is in no way suggested as a substitution of medical and pharmacological guidelines. Some of the drugs described in this manual are not yet supported by evidence-based medicine for their efficacy against COVID-19 and cautions therefore must be taken in applying the contents to clinical practice.

This manual is prepared for timely matter based on limited information and time, and thus limitations are inevitable. Suggestions and criticisms will be greatly appreciated.

Yang Baofeng

March 3, 2020

目 录

Contents

Contents

第一部分

具有抗病毒作用的药物

阿比多尔

阿比多尔（arbidol）是一种非核苷类的广谱抗病毒药物。

【体内过程】

阿比多尔口服吸收迅速，1.38h后血药浓度达峰值，血浆蛋白结合率高达90%。阿比多尔经肝脏代谢、胆汁排泄，$t_{1/2}$为15.7h。阿比多尔在体内分布广泛，在肝脏中浓度最高。

【药理作用及机制】

阿比多尔是一种广谱抗病毒药物，通过抑制病毒的侵入（即脂膜与宿主细胞的融合）从而阻断病毒的复制。大量研究显示，阿比多尔对多种病毒［甲型流感病毒、乙型流感病毒、呼吸道合胞病毒、柯萨奇病毒、中东呼吸综合征冠状病毒（MERS-CoV）、严重急性呼吸综合征冠状病毒（SARS-CoV）、腺病毒、乙型肝炎病毒和丙型肝炎病毒等］均具有抑制作用。阿比多尔还可诱导内源性干扰素的产生和释放，激活巨噬细胞参与免疫调节。目前体外试验显示，阿比多尔有显著的抗新型冠状病毒作用。

【临床应用】

1. 可用于预防和治疗由甲、乙型流感病毒引起的上呼吸道感染。

2. 是用于治疗中东呼吸综合征(MERS)和严重急性呼吸综合征(SARS)相关冠状病毒感染的专利药物。

3.《新型冠状病毒肺炎诊疗方案(试行第七版)》中推荐阿比多尔作为抗新冠肺炎治疗药物。

【用法用量】

《新型冠状病毒肺炎诊疗方案(试行第七版)》推荐阿比多尔剂量为成人 200mg,每日 3 次,疗程不超过 10d。

【不良反应】

主要表现为恶心、腹泻、头晕和血清转氨酶增高。

【药物相互作用】

阿比多尔的血浆蛋白结合率高达 90%,与某些蛋白结合率高的药物联用会产生对血浆蛋白的竞争性结合,导致外周血中游离型的阿比多尔浓度显著升高,在临床上应及时调整阿比多尔的给药剂量。

干 扰 素

干扰素(interferons,IFNs)是机体受到病毒的感染刺激后,体内的单核细胞和淋巴细胞产生的一类具有抗病毒作用的糖蛋白物质,具有广谱抗病毒作用。

【药理作用及机制】

IFNs 抗病毒作用广泛,除了能阻断病毒侵入、扩增、释放等各阶段外,对病毒的再次感染和病毒的持续性感染也有一定阻碍作用。大多数细胞在病毒感染后均能产生 IFN-α 和 IFN-β 两种亚型的 IFNs,IFN-α 和 IFN-β 主要通过刺激淋巴细胞、自然杀伤细胞和巨噬细胞等免疫细胞发挥其较强的抗病毒作用;而 IFN-γ 这种亚型仅由 T 淋巴细胞和自然杀伤细胞生成与释放,所以 IFN-γ 的抗病毒作用较弱,但在免疫调节方面具有明显的调控作用。

病毒根据种类的不同,它们在侵入、脱壳、细胞内扩增、病毒颗粒组装和释放等各阶段都有各自的特点。IFNs 在不同病毒中的作用靶点及机制也各有不同,对不同病毒的抗病毒效果也有较大差异。当 IFNs 进入细胞后能够诱导蛋白激酶、寡腺苷酸合成酶、核糖核酸酶等的表达,从而发挥其抗病毒作用。早在 2013 年,瑞士科学家就发现某些种类的 IFNs 能抑制冠状病毒在人类呼吸道上皮细胞中的复制。同时在体外研究中也发现 IFN-α 以及 IFN-β 对 MERS-CoV 和 SARS-CoV 具有较强的抗病毒效果。这些研究成果为 IFNs 在本次新冠肺炎的临床应用提供了理论基础。

【临床应用】

1. 抗病毒作用　IFNs 是一类广谱抗病毒药,临床上主要用于各种急性病毒感染性疾病(包括流感、病毒性心肌炎、流行性腮腺炎、乙型脑炎等)和慢性病毒性感染(如慢性活动性乙型肝炎、巨细胞病毒感染等)。

2. 抗肿瘤作用　IFNs 通过抑制肿瘤细胞的增殖和调节患者免疫功能来发挥其抗肿瘤作用。目前,IFNs 已经广泛用于肿瘤治疗。

3. 抗新冠肺炎作用　《新型冠状病毒肺炎诊疗方案(试行第七版)》中推荐 α-干扰素作为抗新冠肺炎治疗药物。

【用法用量】

《新型冠状病毒肺炎诊疗方案(试行第七版)》推荐试用 α-干扰素,剂量为成人每次 500 万 U 或相当剂量,加入灭菌注射用水 2ml,每日 2 次雾化吸入。

【不良反应】

1. IFNs 最常见的不良反应为流感样综合征,患者用药后常会出现一过性发热、寒战、食欲缺乏、头痛、肌肉酸痛、乏力、恶心、呕吐。

2. 少数患者在用药后会出现骨髓抑制、肝功能异常、肾脏损害等一过性损害，但停药后症状即消失。

3. 在 IFNs 使用过程中应重视其对中枢和外周神经系统的毒副作用，如乏力、嗜睡、情感淡漠、抑郁、重度焦虑等，患有精神疾病的患者应禁用。

氯　喹

氯喹（chloroquine）是人工合成的 4-氨基喹啉类衍生物。磷酸氯喹是氯喹的磷酸盐，成盐的目的是提高药物稳定性和溶解性。

【体内过程】

氯喹口服吸收迅速而完全，1~2h 后血药浓度达峰值，血浆蛋白结合率为 55%。氯喹在体内分布范围广，可以透过红细胞膜并在红细胞内部蓄积，当红细胞被疟原虫侵入后，氯喹在其中的浓度进一步升高，这为氯喹抗疟疾提供了重要保障。氯喹经肝脏代谢，$t_{1/2}$ 为 50h；经肾脏排泄，酸化尿液可促进其排泄，这可用于氯喹中毒时的解救。

【药理作用及机制】

氯喹能够杀灭疟原虫在红细胞内的裂殖体，其作用机制为抑制疟原虫裂殖体 DNA 的复制、转录与翻译；但氯喹对静止期的子孢子、休眠子和配子体无抑制作用，因此氯喹不能抑制疟疾的传播。氯喹在肝脏中的药物浓度显著高于血药浓度，能显著杀灭定植于肝脏的阿米巴滋养体。目前在多中心临床研究中发现磷酸氯喹对新冠肺炎有一定的疗效。

【临床应用】

1. **抗疟疾作用**　氯喹可以迅速有效地控制疟疾的发作，进入疫区后预防性给药能抑制疟疾临床症状发作。

2. **预防性给药**　氯喹能预防性抑制疟疾症状发作，

在进入疫区前 1 周和离开疫区后 4 周期间,每周服药一次即可。

3. 抗肠道外阿米巴病　临床上用于治疗阿米巴肝脓肿患者。

4. 抗病毒作用　对多种病毒有抑制作用。

5. 免疫抑制　大剂量氯喹和羟氯喹能抑制体内免疫反应,因此临床上使用硫酸羟氯喹来治疗系统性红斑狼疮等自身免疫性疾病。

6. 抗新冠肺炎作用　《新型冠状病毒肺炎诊疗方案(试行第七版)》中推荐磷酸氯喹作为抗新冠肺炎治疗药物。

【用法用量】

磷酸氯喹用于新冠肺炎的治疗仅适用于 18~65 岁成人。具体用法用量为:体重大于 50kg 者,每次 500mg、每日 2 次,疗程 7 日;体重小于 50kg 者,第一、二日每次 500mg、每日 2 次,第三至第七日每次 500mg、每日 1 次。并且在使用过程中应根据患者体重等差异调整磷酸氯喹的用法用量。

【不良反应】

1. 大剂量使用氯喹可发生恶心、呕吐、头晕、过敏等不良反应,餐后服用可有效减少副作用的发生。

2. 长时间使用时可导致视力障碍、视网膜水肿,长期使用氯喹的患者应定期进行眼科相关检查。已知患有视网膜疾病的患者禁用。

3. 氯喹经静脉快速给药时,可致患者血压降低;大剂量氯喹还可抑制窦房结,严重者可致阿 - 斯综合征甚至死亡,患有心脏疾病的患者禁用。在国家卫生健康委员会发布的《关于调整试用磷酸氯喹治疗新冠肺炎用法用量的通知》中指出,使用磷酸氯喹治疗新冠肺炎的患者,用药前必须心电图检查正常,禁止同时使用喹诺酮类、大环内酯类抗生素及其他可能导致 QT 间期延长的药物。

4. 氯喹可损害听力,孕妇大量服用氯喹后可造成小儿先天性耳聋、智力迟钝等,处于妊娠期女性禁用,听力减退或听力丧失的患者禁用。

5. 葡萄糖 -6- 磷酸脱氢酶缺乏者服用氯喹可发生溶血性贫血,葡萄糖 -6- 磷酸脱氢酶缺乏症患者禁用。

【药物相互作用】

1. 磷酸氯喹与链霉素合用能够加重对神经肌肉接头的抑制作用。

2. 与洋地黄合用能够抑制心脏电传导,从而产生心脏毒性。

3. 与肝素或青霉胺合用可增加出血概率。

4. 与喹诺酮类、大环内酯类抗生素及其他可能导致 QT 间期延长的药物合用时可使 QT 间期进一步延长,导致恶性心律失常的发生。

【禁忌证】

国家卫生健康委员会发布的《关于调整试用磷酸氯喹治疗新冠肺炎用法用量的通知》中明确规定了磷酸氯喹的如下禁忌证:处于妊娠期的女性患者;明确对 4- 氨基喹啉类化合物过敏的患者;患有心律失常(如传导阻滞)、慢性心脏病的患者;患有慢性肝、肾疾病并达到终末期的患者;已知患有视网膜疾病、听力减退或听力丧失的患者;已知患有精神类疾病的患者;皮肤疾病(包括皮疹、皮炎、银屑病)患者;葡萄糖 -6- 磷酸脱氢酶缺乏症患者;因原有基础疾病必须使用洋地黄类药物、保泰松、肝素、青霉胺、胺碘酮、卞普地尔、多潘立酮、氟哌利多、氟哌啶醇、阿奇霉素、阿司咪唑、红霉素、克拉霉素、泊沙康唑、美沙酮、普鲁卡因胺、氢氯噻嗪、斯帕沙星、左氧氟沙星、莫西沙星、西沙比利、吲达帕胺、氯丙嗪、链霉素、青霉胺、氯化铵、昂丹司琼、阿扑吗啡、奥曲肽单胺氧化酶抑制剂、氟羟强的松龙等药物的患者。

利巴韦林

利巴韦林（ribavirin，virazole，三氮唑核苷，病毒唑）是一种人工合成的鸟苷类衍生物，为广谱抗病毒药物。

【体内过程】

利巴韦林可通过口服、气溶胶、眼部房水等多种途径被吸收进入体内。其口服吸收迅速，生物利用度约为 45%，并在口服 1.5h 后血药浓度达峰值。利巴韦林经肝脏代谢，经肾脏排泄，药物 $t_{1/2}$ 为 0.5~2h。

【药理作用及机制】

利巴韦林为广谱强效抗病毒药，对多种 RNA 和 DNA 病毒（如呼吸道合胞病毒、疱疹病毒、流感病毒、甲型肝炎病毒、丙型肝炎病毒、汉坦病毒、腺病毒等）均具有抑制作用。当利巴韦林进入被病毒感染的细胞后能够迅速被磷酸化，其磷酸化产物可以作为病毒合成酶的竞争性抑制剂，抑制在病毒复制过程中的多种关键酶，从而抑制病毒 RNA 的复制和蛋白质合成，最终使病毒的增殖与释放受到抑制。利巴韦林不能影响病毒吸附、注入和脱壳的过程，同时也不能诱导体内干扰素的产生，所以利巴韦林对病毒感染的预防作用较弱。体外试验显示，利巴韦林对冠状病毒有抑制作用。

【临床应用】

1. 用于治疗急性甲型和丙型肝炎。

2. 用于治疗呼吸道合胞病毒肺炎、支气管炎和流感。

3.《新型冠状病毒肺炎诊疗方案（试行第七版）》中推荐利巴韦林作为抗新冠肺炎治疗药物。

【用法用量】

《新型冠状病毒肺炎诊疗方案（试行第七版）》推荐利巴韦林与干扰素或洛匹那韦 / 利托那韦联合应用，剂量为成人

500mg/次,每日 2~3 次静脉输注,疗程不超过 10d。

【不良反应】

1. 利巴韦林能够在红细胞内大量蓄积,因此常见的不良反应为贫血、乏力等,停药后症状即消失。

2. 动物实验显示利巴韦林有致癌、致畸和致突变作用,且可透过胎盘屏障,也能进入乳汁,孕妇及哺乳期妇女禁用。

3. 有病例显示贫血的患者服用利巴韦林可引发心肌损害,有心脏病病史的患者应慎用。

【药物相互作用】

利巴韦林可抑制齐多夫定向磷酸齐多夫定的转化,二者合用会产生拮抗作用。在治疗丙型肝炎时利巴韦林与干扰素联合应用可产生协同作用。大剂量使用利巴韦林会产生严重的不良反应,在《新型冠状病毒肺炎诊疗方案(试行第七版)》中建议将利巴韦林与干扰素或洛匹那韦/利托那韦合用,从而产生协同作用,降低利巴韦林的使用剂量,增加抗病毒活性,减少不良反应。

HIV 蛋白酶抑制剂

HIV 蛋白酶抑制剂包括利托那韦(ritonavir)、奈非那韦(nelfinavir)、沙奎那韦(saquinavir)、茚地那韦(indinavir)、安普那韦(amprenavir)和洛匹那韦(lopinavir)等。

【药理作用及机制】

蛋白酶是 HIV 复制过程中的关键酶,能够催化 HIV 蛋白前体裂解,促进结构蛋白的形成和 HIV 病毒的成熟、释放。而蛋白酶抑制剂则可阻止前体蛋白的裂解,抑制未成熟的非感染性病毒颗粒的进一步活化,并最终产生抗病毒作用。

冠状病毒的复制与 HIV 病毒的复制类似,也需要病毒蛋白酶的催化。前期体外研究显示洛匹那韦和利托那韦等能够显著抑制 MERS-CoV 以及 SARS-CoV 的复制,洛匹那韦和利托那韦具有抗冠状病毒的潜力。

【临床应用】

1. 治疗成人的 HIV 感染时,可与核苷类反转录酶抑制剂类或非核苷类反转录酶抑制剂类联合使用,从而产生协同作用。

2. 对于在临床上不适宜使用核苷或非核苷类反转录酶抑制剂治疗的成年 HIV 患者,可以单独应用蛋白酶抑制剂进行治疗。

3.《新型冠状病毒肺炎诊疗方案(试行第七版)》中推荐利托那韦和洛匹那韦作为抗新冠肺炎治疗药物。

【用法用量】

《新型冠状病毒肺炎诊疗方案(试行第七版)》推荐洛匹那韦 / 利托那韦的剂量为成人 200mg/50mg/ 粒,每次 2 粒,每日 2 次,疗程不超过 10d。

【不良反应】

1. **神经系统反应**　眩晕、头痛、感觉及反应迟钝、失眠、味觉异常。

2. **胃肠道反应**　食欲不振、厌食、恶心、呕吐、腹痛、腹泻。

3. **过敏反应**　药物热、皮肤干燥、瘙痒、药疹、皮肤红斑。

4. **肝、肾功能异常。**

5. **血液系统反应**　自发性出血、溶血性贫血。

6. **代谢反应**　胰岛素抵抗、高血糖、高血脂。

【药物相互作用】

蛋白酶抑制剂主要经肝细胞色素 P450 代谢,可与其他许多抑制细胞色素 P450 酶的药物发生相互作用,从而降低药效。某些蛋白酶抑制剂在体内的生物利用度是随体内 pH 的改变而改变,当其与抗酸剂、H_2 受体拮抗剂及质子泵抑制剂合用时,可导致蛋白酶抑制剂的血浆浓度下降。

法匹拉韦

法匹拉韦(favipiravir)是一种 RNA 依赖的 RNA 聚合酶抑制剂。

【体内过程】

法匹拉韦口服吸收良好,生物利用度高。法匹拉韦在外周血中的血浆蛋白结合率为 53%,分布广泛。法匹拉韦经肝脏代谢、经肾脏排泄。

【药理作用及机制】

法匹拉韦在体内可迅速转化为法匹拉韦核苷三磷酸(M6)形式,M6 通过模拟鸟苷三磷酸竞争性抑制病毒 RNA 依赖的RNA 聚合酶,抑制病毒基因组的复制、转录和增殖。M6 还可插入病毒基因组中,通过诱导病毒基因组中核苷酸突变而发挥抗病毒作用。目前体外试验显示,法匹拉韦对新型冠状病毒有显著的抑制作用。

【临床应用】

目前日本已批准法匹拉韦用于新发或复发流感的治疗,美国正在进行其针对流感的Ⅲ期临床研究。有研究显示法匹拉韦对诸多 RNA 病毒(例如埃博拉病毒、黄热病病毒、肠道病毒等)具有很好的抗病毒作用。目前在我国法匹拉韦刚刚获得药品注册批件并投入生产,其适应证是流感,同时批准了该药物作为新冠肺炎的临床试验用药。

【不良反应】

法匹拉韦可引起血尿酸增加、腹泻、中性粒细胞减少、肝脏转氨酶升高等不良反应。

【药物相互作用】

法匹拉韦与吡嗪酰胺合用可使血液中尿酸水平升高;法

匹拉韦与瑞格列奈合用可增加瑞格列奈的血药浓度。

瑞德西韦

瑞德西韦(remdesivir)是一种核苷类似物前药,属于 RNA 依赖的 RNA 聚合酶抑制剂,具有抗病毒活性。

【药理作用及机制】

瑞德西韦以前药(prodrug)形式进入细胞后,通过三步转化为三磷酸代谢物 NTP 的活化形式与 ATP 竞争,终止病毒的 RNA 转录和扩增过程。在临床前研究中发现瑞德西韦能够通过抑制埃博拉病毒 RdRP 蛋白来影响病毒的复制和繁殖。在动物实验中,瑞德西韦具有对抗 MERS-CoV 和 SARS-CoV 的药理活性。

【临床应用】

具有治疗 MERS、SARS、埃博拉病毒感染和新冠肺炎的潜力。

【不良反应】

本品尚未获批上市,其安全性和有效性尚待被证实。

特力阿扎韦(维)林

特力阿扎韦(维)林活性成分主要为嘌呤核苷(鸟嘌呤)碱基的合成类似物,对含 RNA 的病毒具有广泛的抗病毒作用。

【药理作用及机制】

特力阿扎韦(维)林可以抑制病毒 RNA 的合成与复制。Ⅱ期临床试验发现口服特力阿扎韦(维)林可显著缩短流感主要临床症状(中毒、发热、呼吸道症状)的持续时间,降低流感相关并发症的发生率,减少对症药物的使用。特力阿扎韦(维)林还可治疗许多其他病毒导致的疾病,包括蜱传脑炎。此外,还有研究发现特力阿扎韦(维)林具有潜在的抗埃博拉病毒感染作用。杨宝峰院士新近主持的临床试验发现,特力阿扎韦(维)林对新冠肺炎患者有一定疗效,能够提高新冠肺炎临床改善率,缩短治疗时间,促进肺部炎症吸收,提高核酸转阴率,降低重症转化率,改善患者身体炎症反应及血液高凝状态,降低治疗过程中并发症的发生率,降低合并用药比率,如糖皮质激素的使用率和吸氧支持率。

【临床应用】

流感、蜱传脑炎、埃博拉病毒感染、新冠肺炎。

【不良反应】

1. 过敏反应。

2. 胃肠道反应　气胀、腹泻、恶心、呕吐。

参考文献

[1] BLAISING J,POLYAK S J,PÉCHEUR E I.Arbidol as a broad-spectrum antiviral:an update[J].Antiviral Res,2014,107:84-94.

[2] MOMATTIN H,MOHAMMED K,ZUMLA A,et al.Therapeutic options for Middle East respiratory syndrome coronavirus(MERS-CoV)-possible lessons from a systematic review of SARS-CoV therapy[J].Int J Infect Dis,2013,17(10):e792-798.

[3] CAMERON C E,CASTRO C.The mechanism of action of ribavirin:lethal mutagenesis of RNA virus genomes mediated by the viral RNA-dependent RNA polymerase[J].Curr Opin Infect Dis,2001,14(6):757-764.

[4] FURUTA Y,KOMENO T,NAKAMURA T.Favipiravir(T-705),a broad spectrum inhibitor of viral RNA polymerase[J].Proc Jpn Acad Ser B Phys Biol Sci,2017,93(7):449-463.

[5] 杨宝峰,陈建国. 药理学[M].9 版. 北京:人民卫生出版社,2018.

第二部分

激素类药物

糖皮质激素

糖皮质激素(glucocorticoid, GC)是机体调控应激反应最重要的调节激素之一,也是临床上使用最为广泛且有效的抗炎和免疫抑制首选药物。常见的糖皮质激素类药物有泼尼松、甲泼尼龙、氢化可的松和地塞米松等。

【体内过程】

糖皮质激素口服、注射均可吸收。体内主要在肝脏代谢,与葡萄糖醛酸或硫酸结合后,由尿液排出。肝、肾功能不全者体内糖皮质激素代谢周期明显延长。

【药理作用及机制】

1. 物质代谢 糖皮质激素对体内多种物质代谢均有影响。如促进糖异生,升高血糖;加速蛋白质代谢,促机体负氮平衡;促体脂分解后再分布;减少肾小管对水的重吸收,促钙、磷流失。

2. 抗炎 早期应用糖皮质激素可减轻因毛细血管扩张及通透性改变所引起的淋巴细胞渗出;另外,应用糖皮质激素还可抑制毛细血管和成纤维细胞增生,从而防止粘连和瘢痕形成,减轻炎症后遗症。

3. **免疫抑制**　糖皮质激素通过改变细胞内物质跨膜转运,从而调控淋巴细胞核酸代谢,最终抑制炎症因子生成和释放。

4. **抗休克**　糖皮质激素通过抑制炎症因子产生及稳定溶酶体膜,改善由微循环障碍所引起的休克,改善由血管痉挛引起的心肌供血不全和心肌收缩障碍,提高机体对细菌内毒素的耐受,对外毒素无作用。

【临床应用】

1. **感染或炎症**　对急性中毒性感染并伴有休克的患者,糖皮质激素为首选治疗药物。《新型冠状病毒肺炎诊疗方案(试行第七版)》推荐对氧合指标进行性恶化、影像学进展迅速、机体炎症反应过度激活状态的患者,酌情短期内(3~5 日)使用糖皮质激素,建议剂量不超过相当于甲泼尼龙 $1\sim2mg/(kg\cdot d)$。应用糖皮质激素治疗危重症患者具有较好疗效。但是,在应用糖皮质激素的同时也会给患者带来潜在风险(如继发性感染和骨质疏松等)。用糖皮质激素治疗新冠肺炎,应结合已有各项检测结果,准确评估患者疾病进程,密切监控患者生命体征,积极寻找替代药物或替代疗法。

2. **免疫抑制**　糖皮质激素可作为抑制自身免疫性疾病的首选药物(如风湿性心肌炎等)。辅助治疗过敏性疾病(支气管哮喘和过敏性休克等),预防由器官移植所引起的异体免疫排斥。

3. **抗休克**　用抗生素治疗由细菌引起的中毒性休克时,可合用糖皮质激素类药物。对合并基础疾病感染者,应结合疾病的临床特点,多学科会诊明确治疗方案,慎用糖皮质激素或选择替代药物(疗法)。

4. **替代疗法**　用于急 / 慢性肾上腺皮质功能不全或肾上腺皮质激素分泌不足的患者。

【不良反应】

1. 医源性肾上腺皮质功能亢进　长期使用糖皮质激素极易引起机体物质代谢紊乱。常表现为满月脸、水牛背、水肿、低血钾和高血压等。

2. 诱发或加重感染　糖皮质激素在抑制炎症、减轻症状时,也降低了机体的防御和修复功能,有导致感染扩散和延缓创口愈合的风险。

3. 骨质疏松　糖皮质激素长期应用常伴有成骨细胞活力下降,骨基质分解,骨盐沉积障碍,最终诱发骨质疏松,出现骨质疏松时必须停止糖皮质激素使用。用糖皮质激素时应密切监控血清钙/磷含量、每日尿钙/肌酐比值、骨更新标记物改变(如骨钙素、尿吡啶啉和脱氧吡啶啉等),辅以影像学检查骨密度。

4. 糖尿病　长期应用糖皮质激素引起患者体内糖代谢紊乱,出现糖耐量受损和糖尿病。

5. 心肌损伤　长期应用糖皮质激素极易引起机体物质代谢紊乱,诱发高血压和动脉粥样硬化。

6. 消化性溃疡　糖皮质激素可刺激胃酸分泌,降低胃肠黏膜保护,诱发溃疡,长期使用还可造成消化道出血或穿孔。

7. 妊娠　妊娠期妇女应用糖皮质激素可透过胎盘诱发胎儿腭裂畸形或死胎。

8. 癫痫　长期应用糖皮质激素可诱发癫痫或精神失常等中枢神经系统疾病。小儿大剂量应用极易诱发惊厥。

【药物相互作用】

1. 糖皮质激素与非甾体抗炎药合用,减少胃黏液分泌,促蛋白质分解和抑制蛋白质合成,诱发或加重消化性溃疡等疾病。

2. 糖皮质激素与抗抑郁药合用,加重由糖皮质激素所诱发的中枢神经系统疾病。

3. 糖皮质激素与强心苷类合用,诱发的心律失常与糖皮质激素引起的水钠潴留和排钾作用有关。

4. 糖皮质激素引起电解质代谢紊乱,与碳酸酐酶抑制剂合用后,可导致严重低血钾,并且糖皮质激素的水钠潴留作用会减弱利尿药的利尿效应。

5. 糖皮质激素与免疫抑制剂合用,加重感染危险。

6. 蛋白质同化激素与糖皮质激素合用,可增加水肿的发生率,诱发或加重痤疮。

7. 糖皮质激素与抗结核药物联合应用可减少渗出及胸膜粘连。

参考文献

[1] RUSSELL C D,MILLAR J E,BAILLIE J K.Clinical evidence does not support corticosteroid treatment for 2019-nCoV lung injury [J]. Lancet,2020,395(10223):473-475.

[2] 杨宝峰,陈建国.药理学[M].9 版.北京:人民卫生出版社,2018.

第三部分

祛痰药

氯化铵

氯化铵(ammonium chloride)属于恶心性祛痰药的一种。

【药理作用及机制】

该药口服后对胃黏膜产生刺激作用,引起轻度的恶心症状从而刺激迷走神经,反射性地增加呼吸道腺体的分泌,同时其能够升高呼吸道的渗透压,使水分向呼吸道渗出使痰液稀释,便于咳出。

【临床应用】

1. 氯化铵作为恶心性祛痰药可以用于干咳或者黏痰不易咳出者。

2. 亦可用于酸化尿液或是纠正代谢性碱中毒。

【用法用量】

片剂建议用水溶解,饭后服用。

1. **成人用量** 口服:祛痰,一次 0.3~0.6g,一日 3 次;利尿,一次 0.6~2g,一日 3 次。

2. **儿童用量** 每日 30~60mg/kg,或按 $1.5g/m^2$,分 4 次服用。

【不良反应】

1. 口服后可能出现恶心、口渴及呕吐等症状。

2. 过量服用可致高氯性酸中毒、低血钾及低血钠。

【药物相互作用】

1. 与金霉素、新霉素、呋喃妥因、磺胺嘧啶、华法林呈配伍禁忌，且不适宜与排钾利尿药合用。

2. 可促进碱性药物如哌替啶的排泄。

【禁忌证】

1. 对氯化铵过敏者禁用。

2. 严重肝、肾功能不全者，有溃疡病者禁用。

3. 代谢性酸中毒患者禁用。

乙酰半胱氨酸

乙酰半胱氨酸（acetylcysteine）最早应用于 20 世纪 60 年代，是一种经典的黏痰溶解药。

【药理作用及机制】

乙酰半胱氨酸服用吸收后，乙酰半胱氨酸分子中的巯基能使痰液中糖蛋白多肽链中的二硫键以及脓性痰液中的 DNA 纤维断裂，产生较强的黏痰溶解作用，从而有效降低痰液黏度，促进痰液排出，以达到有效治疗目的。

【临床应用】

该药具有较强的黏液溶解能力，一般应用于黏稠分泌物过多为特征的呼吸系统疾病，如急性支气管炎、慢性支气管炎急性发作、支气管扩张症、慢性阻塞性肺疾病等。

【用法用量】

1. **喷雾** 在非紧急情况下使用。临用前，用氯化钠注射液使之溶解成 10% 溶液，喷雾吸入，1~3ml/ 次，2~3 次 /d。

2. **气管滴入** 急救时用 5% 溶液，经气管或直接滴入气管内,1~2ml/次,2~6次/d。

3. 气管注入　急救时,以5%溶液用注射器自气管的甲状软骨环骨膜处注入气管腔内,0.5~2ml/次(婴儿0.5ml/次,儿童1ml/次,成人2ml/次)。

【不良反应】

1. 乙酰半胱氨酸片口服偶尔发生恶心、呕吐、上腹部不适、腹泻、咳嗽等不良反应,一般减量或停药即缓解。罕见皮疹和支气管痉挛等过敏反应。

2. 滴注过快可出现恶心、呕吐、皮疹、瘙痒、支气管痉挛、头晕头痛、发热、过敏反应等、偶可见颜面潮红、血管性水肿、心动过速、红细胞减少、白细胞减少、咽炎、鼻(液)溢、耳鸣。减慢静脉输液滴速可减少不良反应,一般可用抗组胺药物对抗,严重过敏反应患者建议停药处理。直接滴入呼吸道可产生大量痰液,必要时须用吸痰器吸引排痰。

【药物相互作用】

1. 与糜蛋白酶、碘化油、胰蛋白酶属配伍禁忌,严禁合用。

2. 与异丙肾上腺素合用可增强药效,减少不良反应。

3. 与硝酸甘油合用可增强扩血管功能并延缓耐受性,但增加头痛与低血压等不良反应的发生率。

4. 与青霉素类、四环素类、头孢菌素类抗生素合用可减弱青霉素类、四环素类、头孢菌素类的抗菌活性,故该药一般不可与这些药物合用,必要时可间隔4小时交替使用。

5. 与酸性较强药物合用可使本品作用明显降低。

溴己新

溴己新(bromhexine)是一类黏痰调节药,能够降低黏痰的吸附力。

【药理作用及机制】

该药具有较强的黏痰溶解作用,服药吸收后可直接作用于气管、支气管黏膜的黏液产生细胞,使痰中的多糖纤维素裂解,稀化痰液。抑制杯状细胞和黏液腺体合成糖蛋白使痰液中的唾液酸减少,降低痰黏度,同时也能促进纤毛运动,利于痰液排出。

【临床应用】

溴己新具有溶解黏痰的作用,一般应用于慢性支气管炎、肺气肿、哮喘、支气管扩张、硅肺等不易咳出黏痰的患者。脓性痰患者需合用抗生素控制感染。

【用法用量】

1. **口服** 8~16mg/ 次,2~3 次 /d。

2. 皮下注射、肌内注射、静脉注射或静脉滴注:4~8mg/ 次,1~2 次 /d。

3. **雾化吸入** 0.2%,2ml/ 次,1~3 次 /d。

【不良反应】

1. 轻微不良反应可表现为偶有恶心、胃部不适。少数病人可能出现血清转氨酶暂时升高,但可自行缓解。

2. 严重时可出现皮疹、遗尿等。

【药物相互作用】

可增加阿莫西林、红霉素等在黏液中的穿透性和浓度,临床联合使用可增强抗感染治疗效果。

【注意事项】

1. 对该药过敏者禁用。

2. 胃溃疡及孕妇、哺乳期妇女慎用。

3. 儿童必须在成人监护下使用,该药应置于儿童接触不到的地方。

4. 建议在饭后服用。

清肺化痰丸

【主要成分】

酒黄芩、苦杏仁、瓜蒌子、川贝母、胆南星(砂炒)、法半夏(砂炒)、陈皮、茯苓、麸炒枳壳、蜜麻黄、桔梗、白苏子、炒莱菔子、款冬花、甘草。

【药理作用及机制】

桔梗具有宣肺、祛痰、利咽、排脓的功效,对咳嗽痰多、胸闷不畅、咽喉肿痛、失音、肺痈吐脓等症状有作用。黄芩主要成分为黄芩苷,具有清热解毒、清热燥湿、解痉的功效,对温热症、上呼吸道感染、肺热咳嗽等有效。胆南星可清热化痰、息风定惊。苦杏仁主要成分为苦杏仁苷,具有镇咳平喘、抗炎镇痛、润肠通便的作用,对咳嗽气喘、胸满痰多、血虚津亏有效。麻黄主要成分为麻黄碱,具有发汗、平喘、利尿等功效,可用于外感风寒所致的发热、头痛、身痛等表证的缓解。陈皮,理气健脾、调中化痰。款冬花对肺虚久咳不止尤为有效。本药各味中药材合理配伍可降气化痰,止咳平喘。

【适应证】

用于肺热咳嗽,痰多作喘,痰涎壅盛,肺气不畅。

【不良反应】

尚未见报道。

【药物相互作用】

本品中含有麻黄成分,麻黄主要成分为麻黄碱,与其他药物配伍应用时,可发生药物反应。

1. 与桂枝相须为用可增强发汗解表。

2. 与含鞣质成分的药物联合使用会使麻黄碱发生沉淀反应,降低药效。

3. 与铁剂药物合用会产生络合反应,降低铁剂疗效。

4. 与帕吉林等单胺氧化酶抑制药合用会造成高血压危象。

5. 与降血压药物合用可降低降压药物的疗效。

6. 与镇静催眠药合用降低后者疗效。

7. 与阿司匹林等解热镇痛药合用可致大汗虚脱。

8. 与异烟肼合用可致排尿困难。

【注意事项】

1. 服用本品期间应忌食辛辣、油腻食物。

2. 支气管扩张、肺脓疡、肺心病、肺结核患者应在医师指导下服用。

3. 服药期间,若患者服用 3d 病证无改善,或出现高热,或出现喘促气急者,或咳嗽加重,痰量明显增多者应到医院就诊。

4. 儿童、孕妇、体质虚弱及脾胃虚寒者慎用。

5. 本品含有黄芩成分,经临床验证为易致敏药材,对该成分有过敏史者禁用,过敏体质者慎用。

6. 运动员慎用。

参考文献

陆丽娜,董加花,左艳华,等.RP-HPLC 法同时测定清肺化痰丸中 4 种成分[J].中成药,2016,38(09):1956-1959.

祛痰灵口服液

【主要成分】

鲜竹沥,鱼腥草。

【药理作用及机制】

祛痰灵口服液能够通过促进腺体分泌、稀释痰液、加快支气管内皮纤毛运动而起到化痰、排痰的作用;具有镇咳作用,能够减少咳嗽次数。对金黄色葡萄球菌、表皮葡萄球菌和肺炎球菌抑制效果较明显;能够通过增强巨噬细胞吞噬功能和淋巴细胞反应性提高机体免疫力;还具有抗炎作用。所含鱼腥草对于流感病毒、单纯疱疹病毒 -1(HSV-1)、人类免疫缺陷病毒 -1(HIV-1)、严重急性呼吸综合征病毒(SARS-CoV)具有抑制作用,此外鱼腥草还具有镇痛、利尿和抗氧化的作用。

【适应证】

祛痰灵口服液具有清热解毒、化痰止咳的功效。多用于缓解痰热咳嗽,表现为咳嗽、痰多,痰黄黏稠,咯痰不畅,临床用于治疗急、慢性支气管炎,肺炎见上述症候者。

【不良反应】

不良反应不常见且较轻微,主要为气促、喉头水肿、胸闷、心悸、皮疹等,鲜竹沥和鱼腥草性微寒,少数儿童使用本品可出现大便稀薄、次数略增等现象。

【药物相互作用】

本品所含竹沥与生姜汁配伍,宜于痰热之证,能够减轻竹沥的寒胃滑肠之弊。

【注意事项】

1. 对本品过敏者禁用,过敏体质者慎用。

2. 孕妇、体质虚弱者慎用。

3. 本品性寒凉,寒性的痰咳、脾虚便溏者不宜服用。

4. 若患者在服药期间出现 38℃及以上发热,或出现明显气促、喘息、咳嗽加重、痰量增多等症状,应停用本品,到医院就诊。

参考文献

[1] 洪毅明,陈长勋,金若敏,等.祛痰灵口服液药理作用的实验研究

［J］.上海中医药杂志,1996,06：43-46.

［2］梁明辉.鱼腥草的化学成分与药理作用研究［J］.中国医药指南,
2019,02：153-154.

［3］李洁,郑小松.基于网络分析的鱼腥草毒性作用机制［J］.沈阳药
科大学学报,2019,36(11):1047-1055.

［4］许舜根,李茂柏.祛痰灵口服液治疗小儿肺热痰咳150例小结［J］.
上海中医药杂志,1994,12：28.

化痰橘红口服液

【主要成分】

化橘红、百部(蜜炙)、茯苓、半夏(制)、白前、甘草、苦杏仁、
五味子。

【药理作用及机制】

化橘红、半夏、茯苓、甘草理气燥湿化痰;百部润肺止
咳;苦杏仁、白前宣肺降气,化痰止咳;五味子益气敛收。化
橘红具有镇咳、祛痰、抗炎、抑菌作用,可化痰理气、健脾消
食,适于胸中痰滞,咳嗽气喘,饮食积滞,呕吐呃逆等症。百
部具有抗菌、止咳、杀虫、抗病毒等作用。茯苓用于痰饮咳
嗽,痰湿入络,肩背酸痛。半夏具有燥湿化痰,降逆止呕作
用。白前具有降气,消痰,止咳的功效,用于肺气壅实,咳嗽
痰多,胸满喘急。甘草具有清热解毒、治疗咳嗽痰多、补脾
益气等功效。苦杏仁主要成分为苦杏仁苷,具有镇咳平喘、
抗炎镇痛、润肠通便的作用,对咳嗽气喘、胸满痰多、血虚津
亏有效。

【适应证】

理气化痰,润肺止咳。用于痰浊阻肺所致的咳嗽、气喘、
痰多,及感冒、支气管炎、咽喉炎见上述证候者。

【不良反应】

尚未见报道。

【禁忌】

风热者忌用。

【药物相互作用】

如与其他药物同时使用可能会发生药物相互作用,详情请咨询医师或药师。

【注意事项】

1. 服用本品期间应忌烟、酒及辛辣、生冷、油腻食物。

2. 不宜在服药期间同时服用滋补性中药。

3. 服药期间,若患者发热体温超过38.5℃,或出现喘促气急者,或咳嗽加重、痰量明显增多者应去医院就诊。

4. 支气管扩张、肺脓疡、肺心病、肺结核患者出现咳嗽时应去医院就诊。

5. 糖尿病患者及有高血压、心脏病、肝病、肾病等慢性病严重者应在医师指导下服用。

6. 儿童、孕妇、哺乳期妇女、年老体弱者应在医师指导下服用。

7. 服药 3d 症状无缓解,应去医院就诊。

8. 对本品过敏者禁用,过敏体质者慎用。

9. 本品性状发生改变时禁止使用。

10. 儿童必须在成人监护下使用。

参考文献

[1] 戴敬,冯丽,孙明,等.HPLC法测定橘红化痰丸中吗啡的含量[J].药物分析杂志,2008,28(10):1757-1759.

[2] 司徒伟良,陈琳,李海斌,等.RP-HPLC法测定橘红化痰丸中柚皮苷的含量[J].广东药科大学学报,2015,31(1):43-45.

[3] 王艳慧,黄洁文,江晓,等.橘红痰咳液止咳化痰平喘抗炎作用的药效学研究[J].世界科学技术-中医药现代化,2017,19(8):1375-1380.

第四部分

中药

金花清感颗粒

金花清感颗粒是 2009 年甲型 H1N1 流感暴发后由我国中医专家研制的用于抗流感病毒的药物。其以经典名方"麻杏石甘汤"及"银翘散"为基础方,对甲型流感治疗有效。

【主要成分】

金银花、石膏、麻黄(蜜炙)、苦杏仁、黄芩、连翘、浙贝母、知母、牛蒡子、青蒿、薄荷、甘草等。

【药理作用及机制】

金花清感颗粒中的基础方剂"麻杏石甘汤"是张仲景专为清肺热之证设计,麻黄入肺经,具有散肺热的功效,配以具有寒凉之性的石膏温和药性。另其加之以"银翘散"方剂,金银花、连翘清热解毒,薄荷辛散表邪,辅以牛蒡子、甘草调和诸药。对于肺热引起的咳嗽、气喘有较好的疗效。

【适应证】

用于外感湿邪引起的发热,恶寒轻或不恶寒,咽红咽痛,鼻塞流涕,口渴,咳嗽或咳而有痰,舌质红,苔薄黄,脉数等。研究发现,金花清感颗粒治疗流行性感冒风热犯肺证安全有效,《新型冠状病毒肺炎诊疗方案(试行第七版)》推荐为医学观察期乏力伴发热患者用药。

【不良反应】

可见恶心、呕吐、腹泻、胃部不适、食欲减退等胃肠道不良反应。偶见用药后肝功能异常,心悸或皮疹。

【药物相互作用】

金花清感颗粒中所含麻黄与消炎镇痛药合用对胃有刺激性,易加重胃肠道不良反应。麻黄与强心苷类药物合用,可使心肌兴奋性加强,心输出量增加,心率加快。麻黄与肾上腺素合用可促进血管收缩,诱发高血压。

【注意事项】

1. 服用本品期间患者应忌辛辣、生冷、油腻食物,提倡清淡饮食以配合药物发挥作用。

2. 本品含有麻黄,其主要成分为麻黄碱,为拟肾上腺素药,具有缩血管、松弛支气管平滑肌、兴奋中枢的作用,可加重心血管疾病。高血压、心功能不全、青光眼、免疫缺陷者慎用。

3. 本品含有石膏,为寒凉之物,脾胃虚寒者慎用。此外由于麻黄碱的升压作用,妊娠妇女禁用。

4. 肝功能异常的患者服用本品后会导致药物蓄积而中毒,既往有肝脏疾病史或服用本品前肝功能异常者慎用。

5. 本品含有金银花、连翘成分,对本品成分有过敏史者禁用,过敏体质者慎用。

参考文献

李国勤,赵静,屠志涛,等.金花清感颗粒治疗流行性感冒风热犯肺证双盲随机对照研究[J].中国中西医结合杂志,2013,33(12):1631-1635.

藿香正气胶囊(丸、水、口服液)

藿香正气胶囊(丸、水、口服液)是一种临床常用的中成药,主要用于风寒感冒的治疗。

【主要成分】

广藿香、紫苏叶、白芷、白术(炒)、陈皮、法半夏、厚朴(姜制)、茯苓、桔梗、甘草、大腹皮、大枣、生姜。

【药理作用及机制】

藿香具有辟秽、祛湿、和中的作用;紫苏叶具有发表散寒、理气和营、行气宽中、和胃止呕的功效;白术有益气健脾、燥湿利水、止汗的功效;大腹皮能够行气导滞、宽中理气;白芷、茯苓、甘草具有健脾和胃的功效。

现代药理研究发现,藿香正气胶囊(丸、水、口服液)有以下药理作用:

1. **解痉** 藿香正气胶囊、丸、散等均具有抑制胃肠痉挛作用。

2. **镇痛** 藿香正气水在动物实验中对肠系膜损伤引起的内脏躯体反射性疼痛具有镇痛作用。

3. **调节胃肠功能紊乱** 对胃肠动力有双向调节作用,可促进消化吸收,治疗胃胀腹泻,镇吐。促进胃肠损伤修复。

4. **增强细胞免疫功能,抑菌、抗病毒** 对于藤黄八叠球菌、金黄色葡萄球菌、痢疾杆菌及沙门氏菌有抑制作用,并对变形杆菌、红色毛癣菌、石膏样毛癣菌、絮状表皮癣菌、石膏样小孢子菌、白色念珠菌、新型隐球菌、皮炎芽生菌及甲、乙型副伤寒杆菌均有较强的抑菌作用。

5. **抗Ⅰ型变态反应** 藿香正气胶囊抑制变态反应介质释放,可改善过敏体质患者的致敏反应。

【适应证】

用于外感风寒,内伤湿滞,头痛昏重,胸膈痞闷,脘腹胀痛,呕吐泄泻。适用于消化系统、呼吸系统、内分泌系统,儿科、皮肤科、神经内科等疾病的治疗。《新型冠状病毒肺炎诊疗方案(试行第七版)》推荐为医学观察期乏力伴胃肠不适患者用药。

【不良反应】

1. 全身性不良反应 如颜面潮红、双硫仑样反应、过敏反应、低血糖等。

2. 神经系统不良反应 如抽搐、烦躁不安、昏迷、头痛。

3. 心血管系统不良反应 如心悸、心跳加速等。

4. 皮肤不良反应 如药疹、瘙痒等。

5. 其他 还有少见的视觉损害、消化系统及呼吸系统损害等不良反应。

【药物相互作用】

1. 藿香正气胶囊联合左氧氟沙星治疗急性胃肠炎,可加快退热、止泻,缓解腹痛,促进患者临床症状缓解。

2. 加味藿香正气丸与诺氟沙星联合使用治疗急性肠胃炎可改善其临床症状,具有较佳的治疗效果。

3. 藿香正气口服液与氯雷他定联合使用治疗慢性荨麻疹,效果明显,具有良好的安全性。

4. 藿香正气水中含乙醇成分,应避免与头孢类药物同时服用,可导致双硫仑样反应。与镇静催眠药、解热镇痛药同时服用,加重毒性反应。

5. 藿香正气胶囊(丸、水、口服液)中含有藿香、紫苏叶等祛湿、发表散寒药物,服药期间不宜同时服用下列滋补性中药。

补气药:人参、党参、太子参、西洋参、黄芪、山药、甘草等。

补血药:阿胶、枸杞子、何首乌、当归、熟地黄等。

补阴药：百合、麦冬、石斛、天冬、北沙参、南沙参等。

补阳药：冬虫夏草、杜仲、淫羊藿、鹿茸、巴戟天等。

滋补性的中成药包括：人参健脾丸、补中益气丸、杞菊地黄丸、六味地黄丸、乌鸡白凤丸、十全大补丸等。

【注意事项】

1. 有高血压、心脏病、肝病、糖尿病、肾病等慢性病严重者,孕妇或正在接受其他治疗的患者,如需使用本品,均应在医师指导下服用。

2. 小儿、年老体虚者应在医师指导下服用。

参考文献

[1] 李田倪.藿香正气水(滴丸、胶囊、颗粒)致不良反应108例分析[C]//中国药学会医院药学专业委员会.第二十三届全国儿科药学学术会议论文集.2012 :313.

[2] 刘松松,谢益明.101例藿香正气水药品不良反应文献分析[J].中国药物警戒,2017,14(05):317-320.

[3] 王培颖.藿香正气胶囊联合左氧氟沙星治疗39例急性胃肠炎患者的临床研究[J].现代医用影像学,2019,28(05):1186-1187.

[4] 李源.诺氟沙星与加味藿香正气丸联合治疗急性肠胃炎的有效性临床研究[J].首都食品与医药,2019,26(18):67.

[5] 廖剑敏.藿香正气口服液联合氯雷他定治疗慢性荨麻疹的疗效观察[J].中国医药指南,2019,17(32):174-175.

连花清瘟胶囊(颗粒)

连花清瘟胶囊(颗粒)是2003年SARS暴发时研发的抗病毒药物,具有广谱抗病毒的作用。

【主要成分】

连翘、金银花、炙麻黄、炒苦杏仁、石膏、板蓝根、绵马贯众、鱼腥草、广藿香、大黄、红景天、薄荷脑、甘草。

【药理作用及机制】

连花清瘟胶囊（颗粒）主要成分之一连翘性凉味苦，具有解毒消痈之功效，尤治上焦之火，辅以薄荷脑、甘草、清风散热。金银花有抗病原微生物的作用，有清热解毒消炎之功效。鱼腥草具有清热解毒、消痈排脓的作用。连花清瘟胶囊（颗粒）对流行性感冒热毒袭肺证有效。

现代药理研究发现连花清瘟胶囊（颗粒）还具有一定的止咳、化痰和调节免疫力的功能。体外研究表明使用本品不仅对 SARS 病毒有效，还对流感病毒，副流感病毒 1 型，呼吸道合胞病毒，腺病毒 3 型和 7 型，单纯疱疹病毒 1 型和 2 型，金黄色葡萄球菌，甲、乙型溶血性链球菌，肺炎球菌，流感嗜血杆菌等均有一定的抑制作用。连花清瘟胶囊通过抑制 MCP-1（趋化因子，具有促炎作用）表达，从而抑制巨噬细胞向急性放射性肺损伤大鼠肺组织中的聚集，进而减轻炎症反应。连花清瘟胶囊可调控 p38 MAPK 通路，抑制炎症因子释放。

【适应证】

用于治疗流行性感冒属热毒袭肺证，症见：发热或高热，恶寒，肌肉酸痛，鼻塞流涕，咳嗽，头痛，咽干咽痛，舌偏红，苔黄或黄腻等。研究发现连花清瘟胶囊还可用于治疗急性咽炎，用于急性扁桃体炎的配合治疗可缩短其相关症状控制时间。对于急性呼吸道感染、慢性阻塞性肺疾病、病毒性角膜炎、流感、肺炎、手足口病、带状疱疹、咽炎和单纯疱疹也有很好的疗效。《新型冠状病毒肺炎诊疗方案（试行第七版）》推荐为医学观察期乏力伴发热患者用药。

【不良反应】

偶见急性腹泻。少数患者主要表现为胃肠道反应，胃痛、胃部不适，恶心、呕吐、腹胀、腹泻。皮肤系统不良反应，皮疹、瘙痒。

【药物相互作用】

连花清瘟胶囊与头孢呋辛联合应用治疗社区获得性肺炎可以提高治疗效果,缩短患者症状消失时间、住院时间、白细胞恢复时间。连花清瘟胶囊与金荞麦片联合应用治疗甲型H1N1流感,疗效显著、起效快、安全性高。连花清瘟胶囊与美罗培南联合应用,对耐碳青霉烯类鲍氏不动杆菌(CRAB)有协同作用。

【注意事项】

1. 服用本品期间患者应忌烟、酒及辛辣、生冷、油腻食物,提倡清淡饮食以配合药物发挥作用。

2. 本品用于治疗流行性感冒属热毒袭肺证,不适用于风寒感冒,在服药期间不宜同时服用滋补性中药,尤其是温补性中药。

3. 本品含有麻黄,其主要成分麻黄碱有收缩血管、兴奋中枢神经的作用,患有高血压、心脏病的患者应慎用,运动员慎用。

4. 本品含有大黄、石膏等,寒性较强,具有泻火通便的作用,儿童、孕妇、哺乳期妇女、年老体弱及脾虚便溏者应在医师指导下服用。

5. 肝、肾功能不全会导致本品代谢和排泄障碍,发生药物蓄积中毒的现象,患有肝病、糖尿病、肾病等慢性病严重者应在医师指导下服用。

6. 本品含有金银花、连翘、鱼腥草成分,对本品成分有过敏史者禁用,过敏体质者慎用。

参考文献

[1] 雷章,卢宏达,董克臣,等.连花清瘟胶囊抑制急性放射性肺损伤大鼠MCP-1的表达与效应[J].医药导报,2014,33(07):845-849.

［2］张彦芬,唐思文,王海荣,等.连花清瘟胶囊对急性肺损伤小鼠炎症因子的影响[J].食品与药品,2015,17(02):96-99.

［3］冯义.连花清瘟胶囊联合头孢呋辛治疗社区获得性肺炎的临床效果观察[J].名医,2020,(01):236.

［4］郭文明.连花清瘟胶囊联合金荞麦片治疗甲型H1N1流感疗效研究[J].成都医学院学报,2015,10(03):357-359.

［5］史利克,王悦,董星,等.连花清瘟联合美罗培南对耐药菌株的体外抑菌实验[J].中华医院感染学杂志,2019,29(08):1172-1175.

疏风解毒胶囊

疏风解毒胶囊是由湖南的民间秘方"祛毒散"演变而来,由最初的6味中药成分,经研究人员改方添加至8味中药材。通过各类中药材的合理配伍发挥解表、清热解毒的功效,用于时行瘟疫、扁桃体炎、腮腺炎、咽炎、支气管炎、慢性阻塞性肺疾病的治疗。

【主要成分】

虎杖、连翘、板蓝根、柴胡、败酱草、马鞭草、芦根、甘草。

【药理作用及机制】

虎杖药材中的大黄酸、大黄素、白藜芦醇,连翘药材中的松脂素及柴胡中的柴胡皂苷等均有清热解毒之功效,可发挥利胆退黄、祛风利湿的作用;败酱草、板蓝根同样具有清热解毒的作用;甘草则发挥清热调和的作用。

研究发现,疏风解毒胶囊对甲型H1N1流感病毒、呼吸道合胞病毒、单纯疱疹病毒、柯萨奇病毒等均有一定的抑制作用。同时,疏风解毒胶囊可通过减少炎症因子PGE_2及细胞因子水平、进而减少致热介质的产生、增加精氨酸升压素(AVP)的量,发挥解热功效。此外,本品中连翘苷、马鞭草苷、大黄素、毛蕊花糖苷等具有抗炎功效。其机制是降低了血清中PGE_2、IL-1β 和 TNF-α 等炎症因子的水平以及升高 CD4[+]/

$CD8^+$ 和自然杀伤细胞的比例,激活免疫调节过程,进而发挥抗炎作用,对急性咽炎、肺炎链球菌所致的肺炎具有治疗作用。

【适应证】

主治急性上呼吸道感染属风热证,症见:发热,恶风,咽痛,头痛,鼻塞,流浊涕,咳嗽等。可应用于流感、上呼吸道感染等呼吸系统疾病的治疗。同时,疏风解毒胶囊对慢性阻塞性肺疾病患者的气道重塑、过敏性鼻炎-哮喘综合征(风热犯肺证)的鼻部症状具有一定的改善作用;另有研究表明疏风解毒胶囊对寻常型点滴状银屑病、手足口病、带状疱疹等疾病具有积极的治疗效果。《新型冠状病毒肺炎诊疗方案(试行第七版)》推荐为医学观察期乏力伴发热患者用药。

【不良反应】

偶尔有消化道的症状,如恶心、呕吐、腹痛、腹胀等,为小概率事件。偶见过敏性皮疹、头晕、头痛、血压升高、面部红肿、虹膜充血等。

【药物相互作用】

1. 本品与重组人干扰素 α-1b 联合应用治疗小儿疱疹性咽峡炎,可缩短患儿发热时间,加快疱疹消退,减轻疼痛,提高治疗效果。

2. 本品与布地奈德雾化联合应用治疗急性咽炎,可促进临床症状和炎症反应的改善。

3. 本品与盐酸左氧氟沙星片联合应用治疗慢性支气管炎急性发作,可快速缓解临床症状,降低炎症因子水平,具有较好的临床疗效。

【注意事项】

1. 服用本品期间患者应忌烟、酒及辛辣、生冷、油腻食物,提倡清淡饮食以配合药物发挥作用。

2. 本品含有金银花、连翘、板蓝根等成分,对本品成分有过敏史者禁用,过敏体质者慎用。

3. 在使用本品时若需服用其他药物,请先咨询药师。

参考文献

［1］刘静,马莉,陆洁,等.疏风解毒胶囊解热作用机制研究［J］.中草药,2016,47(12):2040-2043.

［2］杨杨,李东野.疏风解毒胶囊联合重组 α-1b 干扰素治疗小儿疱疹性咽峡炎的疗效观察［J］.中国中医急症,2019,28(05):899-900.

［3］朱世明,毛晓萍,刘全.疏风解毒胶囊联合布地奈德雾化治疗急性咽炎(风热证)的临床观察［J］.中国医学创新,2019,16(08):67-71.

［4］尹照萍,孙帅.疏风解毒胶囊联合左氧氟沙星治疗慢性支气管炎急性加重期的临床研究［J］.现代药物与临床,2018,33(11):2880-2883.

防风通圣丸(颗粒)

防风通圣丸(颗粒)原为"防风通圣散",在《黄帝素问宣明论方》中改为丸剂,具有外散风寒、内清里热的双重功效。

【主要成分】

防风、荆芥穗、薄荷、麻黄、大黄、芒硝、栀子、滑石、桔梗、石膏、川芎、当归、白芍、黄芩、连翘、甘草、白术(炒)。

【药理作用及机制】

防风通圣丸(颗粒)具有解表通里,清热解毒的功效。此药中的防风具有解热抗炎、抗菌、增强免疫力的功效;麻黄具有解热、抗炎、镇痛的作用;荆芥穗主要有发热退汗、抗菌消炎、止血、退寒热、消痈等功效与作用;桔梗对皮肤过敏性炎症损伤有显著效果;白芍则起到抗炎的作用。研究发现防风通圣丸可增加慢性特发性荨麻疹患者 $CD4^+/CD8^+$ 的比例,提高细胞免疫功能。

【适应证】

用于外寒内热,表里俱实,恶寒壮热,头痛咽干,小便短赤,大便秘结,风疹湿疮。对肥胖、荨麻疹、痤疮、湿疹、皮炎、瘙痒症、头痛、结膜炎、银屑病、疖肿、哮喘等疾病具有一定疗效。

【不良反应】

偶见皮疹等皮肤过敏反应,或大便次数增多且不成形。停药或减量后可恢复。

【药物相互作用】

防风通圣丸与氯雷他定、地氯雷他定或咪唑斯汀联合治疗慢性荨麻疹有较好的效果,有效降低复发率。防风通圣丸与复方甘草酸苷、维生素 E 联合应用治疗非酒精性脂肪肝,改善患者肝功能和血脂指标,且未见明显不良反应。

【注意事项】

1. 服用本品期间,忌烟、酒及辛辣、生冷、油腻、鱼虾海鲜类食物,提倡清淡饮食。

2. 服药期间不宜同时服用补气、补血、补阳、补阴等滋补性中药。

3. 肝、肾功能不全者会导致药物排泄障碍,发生药物蓄积中毒的现象。

4. 肝病、糖尿病、肾病等慢性病者应在医师指导下服用。

5. 儿童、孕妇、哺乳期妇女、年老体弱及脾虚便溏者应在医师指导下服用。

6. 高血压、心脏病病史者慎用;运动员慎用。

7. 过敏体质者慎用。

参考文献

［1］赵梦,彭玉琴,施京红,等. 防风通圣散治疗慢性荨麻疹研究概况［J］.中国民族民间医药,2017,26(04):45-48.

［2］屈恩荣. 防风通圣丸联合氯雷他定治疗慢性荨麻疹的临床疗效观察［J］.继续医学教育,2019,33(05):156-157.

［3］闫月. 防风通圣丸联合地氯雷他定治疗慢性荨麻疹的临床研究［J］.现代中西医结合杂志,2015,24(35):3945-3947.

［4］温生文,杨振明,吕言,等. 防风通圣丸联合咪唑斯汀治疗慢性荨麻疹疗效观察［J］.临床合理用药杂志,2012,5(07):77-78.

［5］何玉飞. 防风通圣丸联合复方甘草酸苷治疗非酒精性脂肪性肝病临床研究［J］.浙江中西医结合杂志,2019,29,(03):197-200.

双黄连口服液(粉针剂)

双黄连口服液(粉针剂)是由金银花、黄芩、连翘组成的纯中药制剂,具有良好的清热解毒、表里双清的作用。可清热解毒、消肿止痛、广谱抗病毒、抑菌、提高机体免疫功能。

【主要成分】

金银花、黄芩、连翘。

【药理作用及机制】

1. 抗菌作用　双黄连口服液(粉针剂)对金黄色葡萄球菌、变形杆菌、大肠埃希菌、铜绿假单胞菌、肺炎链球菌均有较好的抑制作用。抗菌作用机制主要包括直接破坏细菌的细胞结构、降低内毒素增强免疫防疫、干扰细菌生物膜形成过程、抑制微生物酶活性及抑制细菌外排泵的活性。

2. 抗病毒作用　双黄连口服液具有广谱抗病毒作用,对流感病毒(H7N9、H1N1、H5N1)、SARS-CoV、MERS-CoV、柯萨奇病毒具有明显的抗病毒效应。在新型冠状病毒肺炎疫情发生后,上海药物所联合武汉病毒研究所细胞实验证实了双黄连口服液对该病毒具有抑制作用。双黄连口服液（粉针剂）成分中的黄芩泻火解毒、清肺热，通过增强机体自然杀伤细胞活性发挥抗病毒作用；金银花清热解毒、凉血利咽，提高白细胞吞噬功能，抑制病毒增殖；连翘清热解毒、消肿散结，诱导机体产生干扰素和免疫球蛋白，具有抗病毒作用。

3. 抗炎作用　双黄连口服液（粉针剂）有较强的解热、抗炎作用。通过抑制血管通透性、抑制炎症细胞合成及炎症因子分泌，发挥抗炎作用。

4. 增强免疫力　双黄连口服液（粉针剂）是一种多功能的免疫增强剂，可增强人体细胞和体液免疫功能，在抗感染治疗中具有重要作用；还能够提高淋巴细胞的转化率，增强补体效价从而增强机体的免疫力。

【适应证】

1. 双黄连口服液用于外感风热所致的感冒，症见发热、咳嗽、咽痛。

2. 双黄连口服液对轻型甲型 H1N1 流感、口腔炎、小儿流行性腮腺炎有积极的治疗效果。

3. 双黄连粉针剂用于风温邪在肺卫或风热闭肺证，症见发热，微恶风寒或不恶寒，咳嗽气促，咯痰色黄，咽红肿痛等。适用于病毒和细菌引起的急性上呼吸道感染、急性支气管炎、扁桃体炎、轻型肺炎。

4. 双黄连粉针剂对急性尿路感染、儿童重症流行性腮腺炎、病毒性脑炎、手足口病均有较好的临床疗效。

【不良反应】

本品常见的不良反应包括皮疹、瘙痒、血管神经性水肿、消化系统和神经系统病变。消化系统不良反应为一过性，停药或常规处理即可恢复。静脉给药后易发生呼吸系统、血液系统不良反应，高热、寒战、过敏性休克等。

【药物相互作用】

双黄连口服液联合干扰素雾化吸入治疗小儿疱疹性咽峡炎效果明显，可缩短病程；与利巴韦林合用对轻型甲型H1N1流感有较好的疗效；与青霉素联合治疗小儿呼吸道感染效果较好；在雷尼替丁基础上应用双黄连口服液，短时间内改善患者疼痛症状，促进溃疡愈合，提高免疫功能，临床疗效较好。

双黄连口服液中含有辛凉解表、清热解毒功效的中药，患者在服药期间不宜同时服用下列滋补性中药。

补气药：人参、党参、太子参、西洋参、山药、甘草等。

补血药：阿胶、枸杞子、何首乌、当归、熟地黄等。

补阴药：百合、麦冬、石斛、天冬、北沙参、南沙参等。

补阳药：冬虫夏草、杜仲、淫羊藿、鹿茸、巴戟天等。

滋补性的中成药包括：人参健脾丸、补中益气丸、杞菊地黄丸、六味地黄丸、乌鸡白凤丸、十全大补丸等。

双黄连粉针剂联合地塞米松、α-糜蛋白酶雾化吸入可改善全麻气管插管患者术后呼吸道症状；与阿昔洛韦合用降低病毒性脑炎患者的炎症因子表达水平，达到抗病毒的作用；与头孢吡肟合用导致细胞内头孢吡肟增加，引起细胞受损导致肾毒性增加。双黄连粉针剂与氨基糖苷类（庆大霉素、卡那霉素、链霉素）及大环内酯类（红霉素、吉他霉素）、喹诺酮类等配伍易产生浑浊或沉淀，请勿配伍使用。

【注意事项】

目前尚缺乏双黄连口服液（粉针剂）对新型冠状病毒治疗作用的循证医学证据。

双黄连口服液的注意事项如下：

1. 患者在服药期间应忌烟、酒、辛辣、生冷及油腻食物。

2. 风寒感冒者不适用。

3. 糖尿病、高血压、心脏病、肝病、肾病等慢性病严重者应在医师指导下服用。

4. 儿童、孕妇、哺乳期妇女、年老体弱及脾虚便溏者应在医师指导下服用。

5. 对本品过敏者禁用,过敏体质者慎用。

双黄连粉针剂的注意事项:

1. 用药前认真询问患者对本品的过敏史,高敏体质或对同类产品有过敏史者禁用。

2. 咳喘、严重血管神经性水肿、静脉炎患者、年老体弱者、心肺严重疾病患者应避免使用。

3. 不得超剂量或浓度(建议静脉滴注时药液浓度不应超过 1.2%)应用,尤其是儿童,要严格按体重计算用量。

4. 静脉滴注本品应遵循先慢后快的原则。开始滴注时应为 20 滴 /min,15~20min 后,患者无不适,可改为 40~60 滴 /min,并注意监护患者有无不良反应发生。

5. 本品与生理盐水或 5%~10% 葡萄糖溶液配伍时如出现浑浊或沉淀,请勿使用(本品的最佳配伍 pH 为 6~8)。

6. 首次用药应密切观察,一旦出现皮疹、瘙痒、颜面充血,特别是出现心悸、胸闷、呼吸困难、咳嗽等症状应立即停药,并及时给予脱敏治疗。

参考文献

[1] 郭洁,宋殿荣.双黄连的药理作用和临床应用及不良反应研究进展[J].临床合理用药杂志,2017,10(21):161-163.

[2] 贾静.双黄连口服液的临床应用评价[J].中国医院用药评价与分析,2013,13(02):110-112.

[3] 黄露.双黄连口服液联合青霉素治疗上呼吸道感染疗效观察[J].实用中医药杂志,2018,34(05):563-564.

[4] 邱军成,刁诗光.双黄连粉针与头孢他啶联合应用治疗小儿支气管肺炎疗效分析[J].吉林医学,2014,35(12):2548.

[5] 李安泰,顾乃兵,田晔,等.双黄连注射液对病毒性脑炎炎症因子表达的影响[J].陕西中医,2015,36(09):1109-1110.

葛兰香口服液

葛兰香口服液于2019年上市,其处方选自临床应用多年的验方"五根汤"。葛兰香口服液具有清热解表、通里泻热的功效。现代药理实验证明,葛兰香口服液对小鼠肺内呼吸道感染有关的流感病毒增殖量有显著抑制作用。

【主要成分】

葛根、板蓝根、芦根、北豆根、白茅根、广藿香、红花、大黄。

【药理作用及机制】

1. 抗炎作用 葛兰香口服液具有抗炎作用,抑制毛细血管通透性。

2. 抗病毒作用 对肺内流感病毒增殖具有显著的抑制作用。

3. 抑菌作用 体内对流感杆菌和肺炎克雷伯菌有抑制作用;体外对乙型溶血性链球菌、金黄色葡萄球菌、白念珠菌、肺炎双球菌有抑制作用。

4. 解热作用 对啤酒酵母致大鼠体温升高及三联菌苗致兔体温升高均有抑制作用。

【适应证】

清热解表,通里泻热。用于普通感冒属外感风热兼内有积滞证,症见发热恶寒、头部胀痛、鼻塞流涕、咽红咽痛、口干口渴、腹胀便秘,小便黄赤、舌红苔薄白或黄、脉浮数或滑数。

【不良反应】

偶见胃部不适、腹泻。

【药物相互作用】

不宜在服药期间同时服用下列滋补性中药：

补气药：人参、党参、太子参、西洋参、黄芪、山药、甘草等。

补血药：阿胶、枸杞子、何首乌、当归、熟地黄等。

补阴药：百合、麦冬、石斛、天冬、北沙参、南沙参等。

补阳药：冬虫夏草、杜仲、淫羊藿、鹿茸、巴戟天等。

滋补性的中成药包括：人参健脾丸、补中益气丸、杞菊地黄丸、六味地黄丸、乌鸡白凤丸、十全大补丸等。

【注意事项】

1. 目前尚缺乏葛兰香对新型冠状病毒治疗作用的循证医学证据。

2. 服药期间忌烟、酒及辛辣、生冷、油腻食物。

3. 风寒感冒者不适宜。

4. 糖尿病、高血压、心脏病、肝病、肾病等慢性病严重者应在医师指导下服用。

5. 儿童、孕妇、哺乳期妇女、年老体弱及脾虚便溏者应在医师指导下服用。

6. 本品不宜长期服用，服药 3d 症状无缓解应去医院就诊。

7. 体虚者慎用。

8. 久置后如出现沉淀物，可摇匀后服用。

参考文献

[1] 李滟，董立静，李会霞.五根汤加减在儿科热证中的应用[J].内蒙古中医药，2014，33（04）：67-68.

[2] 郑秀萍.一种中药组合物、其制备方法及其应用：ZL200710130194.7[P].2011-7-27.

金振口服液

【主要成分】

山羊角、平贝母、大黄、黄芩、青礞石、石膏、人工牛黄、甘草。

【药理作用及机制】

山羊角具有清热、镇静、散瘀、止痛等功效,对温热症、热毒炽盛等症状具有较好的治疗效果。平贝母主要成分包括生物碱类、生物碱苷类、多糖以及挥发油等,具有清热润肺、化痰止咳、平喘、降压等作用。大黄的有效成分为蒽醌类、蒽酮类,可攻积导滞、活血化瘀、泻火凉血、清热化湿、解毒消痈。黄芩能够解热消肿,具有广谱抗病毒、抗细菌的作用,对温热症、上呼吸道感染、肺热咳嗽等有效。青礞石有坠痰下气、平肝镇惊的功效,对顽痰胶结、咳逆喘急、烦躁胸闷、惊风抽搐等有治疗作用。石膏辛凉宣肺,清热平喘生津;甘草和中缓急,润肺,解毒,调和诸药。本药各味中药材合理配伍可清热解毒,祛痰止咳。

【适应证】

用于小儿急性支气管炎符合痰热咳嗽者,表现为发热、咳嗽、咳吐黄痰、咳吐不爽、舌质红、苔黄腻等。

【不良反应】

偶见用药后便溏,停药后即可恢复正常。

【药物相互作用】

1. 本品不宜与含乌头类药材的中成药合用。

2. 本品成分大黄不宜与以下药物合用:①核黄酸、烟酸、咖啡因、茶碱等药物;②铁剂、洋地黄等药物;③胃蛋白酶、多酶片等药物;④四环素、利福平、磺胺类药物;⑤维生素 B_1、维生素 B_2、烟酸、维生素 B_6、维生素 C;⑥苯巴比妥、磺胺、青霉素、复方阿司匹林等药物；⑦药用炭、鞣酸蛋白、碱性药物；⑧酚妥拉明，可以拮抗前者的止血作用；⑨氯霉素，可以降低前者的泻下作用；⑩异烟肼，容易形成鞣酸盐沉淀使吸收减少。

3. 本品成分黄芩不宜与洋地黄类强心苷、普萘洛尔和青霉素合用。

4. 本品成分人工牛黄不宜与镇静药、麻醉药、抗惊厥药、水合氯醛、吗啡、苯巴比妥、肾上腺素和阿托品合用。

5. 本品成分石膏不宜与四环素类、左旋多巴类、红霉素、利福平、泼尼松、异烟肼和氯丙嗪等药物合用。

6. 本品成分甘草不宜与含甘遂、大戟、芫花或海藻的中成药及降糖西药合用。

【注意事项】

1. 服用本品期间应忌食辛辣、生冷、油腻食物。

2. 不宜在服药期间同时服用滋补性中药。

3. 脾胃虚弱，大便稀溏者慎用。

4. 风寒闭肺、内伤久咳者不适用。

5. 婴儿及糖尿病患儿应在医师指导下服用。

6. 服药期间，若患者服用三天症状无改善，或出现高热体温超过 38.5℃，应到医院就诊。

7. 对该药本品成分有过敏史者禁用，过敏体质者慎用。

参考文献

李瑾 . 金振口服液临床研究应用进展 [J]. 内蒙古中医药 ,2014,33(08): 118-119.

喜炎平注射液

【主要成分】

穿心莲内酯磺化物。

【药理作用及机制】

喜炎平注射液具有较好的抗病毒效果,对于流感病毒和呼吸道合胞病毒具有抑制作用;具有抗菌作用,能够显著抑制痢疾杆菌、肺炎球菌、伤寒杆菌等革兰氏阳性细菌;对于细菌或病毒感染导致的发热具有解热作用;能够舒张平滑肌,缓解气管和支气管痉挛,具有镇咳作用;同时能够增强多种免疫细胞如中性粒细胞、巨噬细胞的功能,促进免疫球蛋白生成,提高免疫力。

【适应证】

用于支气管炎、扁桃体炎、细菌性痢疾等。有研究报道喜炎平注射液可用于轻症流行性感冒患者,也可联合阿奇霉素治疗支原体肺炎。已被纳入《新型冠状病毒肺炎诊疗方案(试行第七版)》中,作为重型新冠肺炎患者用药,可用于新型冠状病毒单独感染或合并轻度细菌感染的患者。

【不良反应】

不良反应主要集中于皮肤及其附件系统、胃肠系统、心血管系统及神经系统。

1. 过敏反应是喜炎平注射液最常见的不良反应,主要表现为皮肤潮红、皮疹、瘙痒、呼吸困难、憋气、荨麻疹、斑丘疹、血管性水肿等。

2. 诱发寒战、发热、多汗、疼痛、乏力、水肿等全身性不良反应;恶心、呕吐、腹泻、腹痛、腹胀、口干、胃痛等消化系统不良反应。

3. 其他不良反应不常见,包括:胸痛、胸闷、呼吸急促、咳嗽等呼吸系统不良反应;心悸、心动过速、心律失常等心血管系统不良反应;头晕、头痛、眩晕、耳鸣等神经系统不良反应。

4. 喜炎平注射液所致的不良反应经停药或对症处理后即可消失。

【药物相互作用】

喜炎平注射液与注射用头孢类抗生素、注射用维生素 B_6 合用可使注射液的 pH 改变,与注射用阿昔洛韦/注射用更昔洛韦合用时,其主要活性成分磺化物 E 含量显著降低。禁止将喜炎平注射液与其他注射液混合后使用,如需联合使用其他静脉用药,应先使用喜炎平注射液,在换药前要冲洗输液管。

【注意事项】

1. 有过敏史、过敏体质的患者慎用,对穿心莲制剂过敏的患者禁用。

2. 为避免不良反应可能出现的严重后果,75 岁以上老人慎用。

3. 对首次使用喜炎平注射液的患者,应在用药初期密切观察患者用药反应,如发现异常应立即停止用药,采取对应的救治措施。

参考文献

[1] 崔佳,司福国.喜炎平注射液的临床应用研究进展[J].淮海医药,2018,36(03):378-380.

[2] 王志飞,张洪春,谢雁鸣,等.喜炎平注射液治疗呼吸系统感染性疾病临床应用专家共识(成人版)[J].中国中药杂志,2019,44(24):5282-5286.

[3] 赵宜乐,董鹏欣,郑丽英,等.喜炎平注射液的循证安全性评估[J].

药品评价,2017,14(11):5-11,61.

[4] 陈媛媛,谢雁鸣,廖星,等.喜炎平注射液符合说明书适应证用药安全性的系统评价[J].中国中药杂志,2016,41(18):3463-3472.

[5] 曾江,吴洪文,杨志杰.喜炎平注射液临床应用安全性的 Meta 分析[J].临床合理用药杂志,2018,11(22):84-86.

痰热清注射液

【主要成分】

黄芩、熊胆粉、山羊角、金银花、连翘。

【药理作用及机制】

痰热清注射液具有抗炎、抗病毒、祛痰、止咳、解热、镇静、平喘等作用。具有广谱抗病原微生物作用,可抑制肺炎链球菌、乙型溶血性链球菌、金黄色葡萄球菌、流感嗜血杆菌、铜绿假单胞菌等呼吸道病原菌;具有显著的抗病毒作用;可有效减轻肺间质水肿,缓解哮喘患者气道痉挛、精神紧张、呼吸不畅,明显减轻气喘、哮鸣音等症状。

【适应证】

痰热清注射液多用于急性支气管炎、上呼吸道感染、急性肺炎、肺脓肿、肺气肿、肺部真菌感染、慢性阻塞性肺疾病等呼吸系统疾病;也可用于手足口病、麻疹、脓毒血症等。痰热清注射液也是治疗中东呼吸综合征、登革热、H7N9 禽流感病毒感染的推荐用药。现已被纳入《新型冠状病毒肺炎诊疗方案(试行第七版)》中,作为重型和危重型新型冠状病毒感染患者用药,尤其是用于新型冠状病毒感染合并轻度细菌感染患者。

【不良反应】

最常见的不良反应为皮肤及附件损害,表现为皮疹、皮肤瘙痒、荨麻疹、斑丘疹等;呼吸系统不良反应也较常见,如呼吸困难、气短、气促;偶见头晕、恶心、呕吐、心慌、发热、寒战等。

【药物相互作用】

1. 本品与头孢哌酮注射液联合应用于治疗社区获得性肺炎及慢性阻塞性肺疾病急性加重期时,可缩短病程,且无明显不良反应发生。

2. 本品与美罗培南合用治疗肺部感染,可减少美罗培南的不良反应,降低真菌感染的发生率。

3. 本品与左氧氟沙星、庆大霉素、阿米卡星、阿奇霉素注射液体外配伍的稳定性较差,不宜配伍应用。

4. 本品不可与含酸性物质的注射剂合用。

5. 本品与汉防己甲素注射液存在配伍禁忌,不能序贯输注。

【注意事项】

1. 有药物过敏史或过敏体质的人群慎用。

2. 老年伴有肝、肾功能不全者,严重肺源性心脏病伴有心力衰竭者,孕妇,24 个月以下婴幼儿以及有表寒证者禁用痰热清注射液。

3. 儿童使用痰热清注射液的不良反应发生率较低,但对有过敏史的高危儿童应提高警惕,在用药期间应密切观察。

参考文献

[1] 潘佩香.痰热清注射液的药理作用及临床应用[J].临床合理用药杂志,2015,8(17):174-175.

[2] 赵宁波,王东兴,杜学航.痰热清注射液治疗呼吸系统疾病临床应用新进展[J].中国中医急症,2018,27(04):740-742.

[3] 王亮,黄翠云,张凤,等.痰热清注射液上市 15 年内研究现状分析[J].中国中医急症,2020,29(01):36-40.

[4] 王双艳,黄德红,王春国.痰热清注射液致不良反应38例系统分析[J].河南中医,2019,39(02):263-266.

[5] 郑薇,聂红霞,尹乐琴,等.痰热清注射液与汉防己甲素注射液存在配伍禁忌[J].当代护士(上旬刊),2016,(03):79.

醒脑静注射液

【主要成分】

麝香、郁金、冰片、栀子。

【药理作用及机制】

醒脑静注射液由安宫牛黄丸改制而成,具有清热开窍、豁痰解毒的功效,对中枢神经系统、循环系统均具有调节作用。

1. **对中枢神经系统的调节作用** 麝香所含麝香酮可降低血管通透性,清除氧自由基,对抗常压缺氧状态,减少脑缺血再灌注损伤引起的海马组织神经细胞凋亡;麝香还可兴奋呼吸中枢、提高动脉血氧分压、降低二氧化碳分压、改善血气指标;醒脑静抑制炎症因子与血管内皮素的表达,降低血液黏度,改善微循环,保护大脑超微结构;组方中栀子具有脱水、利尿、缓解脑水肿的作用。

2. **心血管保护作用** 醒脑静注射液通过影响肾上腺素受体活性而增强心肌耐缺氧能力;其中所含郁金可协同麝香、冰片开窍通络,具有降血脂及改善血液黏度作用;所含栀子有降压作用,可缓解心肌供血及供氧平衡,修复受损的心肌细胞。

3. **解热作用** 醒脑静注射液具有良好的退热效果,且疗效持久。

【适应证】

用于高热昏迷、急性脑梗死、颅脑损伤、结核性脑膜炎、酒精中毒、蛛网膜下腔出血、癫痫的辅助治疗;已被纳入《新型冠状病毒肺炎诊疗方案(试行第七版)》中,作为重型和危重型新冠肺炎感染患者用药,推荐用于新型冠状病毒感染合并高热伴意识障碍患者。应严格按照本品适应证用药,连续使用不得超过14d。

【不良反应】

醒脑静注射液的副作用多以胸闷、呼吸困难、呼吸加快等呼吸系统不良反应为主;偶见皮疹、荨麻疹、面色潮红等过敏反应,以及寒战、发热、头痛、头晕、恶心、呕吐等。

【药物相互作用】

严禁将醒脑静注射液与其他中药注射剂或西药混合滴注。醒脑静注射液以 5% 葡萄糖注射液配制时,其微粒明显高于 0.9% 氯化钠注射液,故建议选择 0.9% 氯化钠注射液作为稀释溶液。醒脑静注射液在 pH 低的溶液中稳定性差。

【注意事项】

1. 有药物过敏史或过敏体质的人群慎用,首次使用醒脑静注射液的患者,应缓慢滴注药液,密切观察患者使用情况。

2. 肝、肾功能异常者慎用,儿童、老年患者慎用,孕妇禁用。

3. 醒脑静注射液具有活血化瘀的功效,应避免与其他同类药物共同使用。

参考文献

[1] 徐元虎.醒脑静注射液的药理药效学研究与临床应用现状[J].现代中西医结合杂志,2010,19(4):507-509.

[2] 刘毅,黄安奇,周汉辉,等.醒脑静注射液联合尼莫地平治疗蛛网膜下腔出血的临床效果[J].中国当代医药,2019,26(36):93-95,99.

［3］陈兴,吴诗华,文建霞,等.醒脑静注射液辅助治疗结核性脑膜炎临床疗效的系统评价[J].中国医院用药评价与分析,2019,19(12):1430-1434,1440.

［4］曹红磊.高压氧联合醒脑静注射液在重型颅脑损伤患者康复治疗中的应用研究[J].现代医药卫生,2020,36(02):256-258.

［5］陈园,裴光明.醒脑静注射液配伍不同稀释液后不溶性微粒的对比观察[J].湖北中医杂志,2016,38(3):72-74.

血必净注射液

血必净注射液为活血化瘀药,体现了中医抗热毒、瘀毒的温病治疗理论,用于治疗炎症、内毒素导致的严重感染性疾病及其引发的器官功能衰竭。

【主要成分】

红花、赤芍、川芎、丹参、当归。

【药理作用及机制】

血必净注射液具有化瘀解毒的功效。现代药理学表明血必净注射液具有抗内毒素、抗氧化、改善微循环、免疫调节等多种药理作用。血必净注射液可降低内毒素水平,拮抗内毒素诱导的内源性炎症介质释放;可提高机体抗氧化应激能力,减轻器官应激性损伤;能够调节过高或过低的免疫反应,增强机体免疫功能;保护血管内皮细胞,改善微循环,保护和修复应激状态下受损的脏器。

【适应证】

血必净注射液可用于治疗温热类疾病瘀毒互结证,症见发热、喘促、心悸、烦躁。

临床研究表明,血必净注射液具有强效抗内毒素的作用,下调促炎因子水平,提升抗炎因子水平,适用于因感染诱发的全身炎症反应综合征及多器官功能障碍综合征器官功能受损期;血必净注射液可显著提升免疫功能并抑制非特异性免疫功能亢进,用于改善脓毒血症免疫功能紊乱状态;血必净注射液可纠正凝血功能紊乱,改善微循环,提升血氧饱和度,减轻应激状态下的器官衰竭。《新型冠状病毒肺炎诊疗方案(试行第七版)》中指出,新型冠状病毒感染重型、危重型患者常伴有炎症因子升高,推荐血必净注射液作为抗新冠肺炎危重症患者出现全身炎症反应综合征及多器官功能衰竭时的治疗药物;在新冠肺炎重症患者联合使用抗菌药物,亦可有效抑制疾病进展。

【不良反应】

1. 呼吸系统症状 患者可出现气促、胸闷、憋喘等症状,这与本品纯度及杂质残留有关。

2. 皮肤症状 患者可出现皮疹、瘙痒、面部潮红。

3. 偶发消化系统症状和心血管系统症状。

【药物相互作用】

1. 静脉滴注过程中禁止与其他注射剂直接配伍使用。

2. 血必净注射液与某些中成药制剂,如丹参川芎嗪和痹祺胶囊的主要活性成分存在重合,不宜合用。

3. 血必净注射液中含有的丹参酮与抗酸药中的金属离子(Ca^{2+}、Al^{3+}、Mg^{2+})形成金属离子络合物,不宜合用。

4. 血必净注射液中含有的丹参不宜与细胞色素 C、维生素 K、士的宁、麻黄碱、阿托品等药物合用,避免影响药效。

5. 血必净注射液联合乌司他丁配伍治疗重症肺炎,可有效改善肺功能、缓解重症肺炎症状。

6. 血必净注射液联合抗生素治疗重症肺感染时,显著减轻炎症反应,未出现严重药物过敏现象,患者肝肾功能、血尿常规等指标未见异常。

7. 血必净注射液与地塞米松联用能够抑制脓毒血症的炎症反应,改善脓毒血症的临床症状。

【注意事项】

1. 本品含红花,有活血功效,孕妇、生理期女性禁用,凝血功能异常者慎用。

2. 老年患者、肝肾功能异常者慎用。合并其他基础疾病患者,应在医生指导下使用。

3. 用药前应详细询问患者过敏史、有无中药注射液不良反应史,并严格按照适应证使用。一旦出现不良反应,应立即停药并对症治疗。

4. 合并其他基础疾病患者,应在医生指导下使用。

参考文献

[1] 张淑文,孙成栋,文艳.血必净注射液对脓毒症大鼠血清炎症介质及 Th1/2 的影响[J].中国危重病急救医学,2006,18(11):673-676.

[2] 陈建,张勇.血必净注射液对脓毒症患者的炎性反应和凝血功能的影响[J].湖南师范大学学报(医学版),2016,13(2):105-107.

[3] 李志军,孙元莹,吴云良,等.血必净注射液防治家兔应激性脏器损伤的研究[J].中国危重病急救医学,2006,18(2):105-108.

[4] 聂爱蕊,郭中坤,张雨,等.211 例血必净注射液不良反应的文献分析[J].海峡药学,2019,31(11):246-249.

[5] 庞剑锋,潘宣百.血必净与乌司他丁配伍治疗重症肺炎的临床效果[J].中国社区医师,2019,35(9):96-98.

[6] 叶青.血必净联合抗生素治疗 ICU 重症肺感染的临床效果分析[J].中国医疗前沿,2013,8(14):29.

[7] 李承羽,张晓雨,刘斯,等.血必净注射液治疗新型冠状病毒感染的肺炎(COVID-19)证据基础及研究前瞻[J].世界科学技术 - 中医药现代化,2020,22(2):1-6.

热毒宁注射液

【主要成分】

青蒿、金银花、栀子。

【药理作用及机制】

热毒宁注射液具有明显的抗炎、抗病毒、解热镇痛、免疫调节等药理作用。热毒宁注射液可显著抑制流感病毒、埃可病毒、疱疹病毒、EV71 病毒及多种呼吸道病毒株;此外,热毒宁注射液具有明显的抗菌作用,对多种细菌菌株均有明显的抑制作用,如金黄色葡萄球菌、乙型溶血性链球菌、大肠埃希菌、志贺菌属、霍乱弧菌、伤寒杆菌、副伤寒杆菌等,对肺炎链球菌、脑膜炎奈瑟菌、铜绿假单胞菌、结核分枝杆菌亦可有效,可降低金黄色葡萄球菌感染和肺炎克雷伯菌感染动物的死亡率,降低血清炎症因子水平;热毒宁注射液亦可减轻发热,增强免疫功能。

【适应证】

用于外感风热、急性上呼吸道感染、急性支气管炎、肺炎所致的咳嗽、高热、恶寒、头痛、痰黄者。

1. 流感 热毒宁注射液联合奥司他韦或金刚烷胺治疗甲型 H1N1 流感,能降低患者体温,明显缩短退热时间和症状消失时间。

2. 慢性支气管炎 热毒宁注射液联合头孢呋辛可治疗慢性支气管炎。

3. 肺炎 热毒宁注射液联合利巴韦林可治疗小儿病毒性肺炎、支原体肺炎,明显缩短咳嗽、肺部啰音消失时间;热毒宁注射液联合左氧氟沙星治疗社区获得性肺炎,明显减轻呼吸道症状,促进白细胞指标恢复;热毒宁注射液联合保护性通气治疗急性肺功能损伤,可明显升高动脉血氧分压,延缓疾病进程,降低病死率。

4.《新型冠状病毒肺炎诊疗方案(试行第七版)》推荐热毒宁注射液作为抗新冠肺炎治疗药物,用于新型冠状病毒感染合并轻度细菌感染患者。

【不良反应】

1. 热毒宁注射液中含有的挥发油、有机酸类、三萜皂苷类及黄酮类化合物在血液中易形成免疫复合物而引起过敏反应,患者表现为全身发红、瘙痒或皮疹等,严重者可出现过敏性休克。

2. 热毒宁注射液还可引起消化系统反应,表现为腹痛、腹泻、胃痛等,个别患者出现头晕、胸闷、口干、恶心、呕吐,儿童居多。

【药物相互作用】

1. 热毒宁注射液与头孢菌素如头孢唑林、头孢呋辛、头孢曲松和头孢哌酮直接配伍后可见不同程度的外观变化。

2. 与喹诺酮类抗生素如左氧氟沙星、加替沙星、盐酸莫西沙星等直接配伍后稳定性较差。

3. 与阿昔洛韦、氨溴索及甲硝唑直接配伍后有微粒物生成。使用热毒宁注射液时,应避免与其他药物直接接触;如需联用,应以 0.9% 氯化钠溶液冲洗输液管或间隔给药。

4. 热毒宁注射液有效成分(栀子苷、槲皮素、绿原酸)对 CYP 酶的活性有一定的影响,与经 CYP 酶代谢的药物合用时,需调整给药剂量。

【注意事项】

1. 本品可引起过敏反应,对本品过敏者及有中药注射液过敏史者慎用;老人、儿童、孕妇、肝肾功能异常者慎用。

2. 本品可升高直接胆红素及总胆红素水平,既往有溶血(血胆红素轻度增高或尿胆原阳性)者慎用。

3. 临床应用本品时,应询问患者年龄、过敏史,并注意给药剂量、速度和疗程。一旦出现不良反应,应立即停药并对症治疗。

4. 合并其他基础疾病患者,应在医生指导下使用。

参考文献

[1] 罗先才.热毒宁注射液药理作用、临床应用及不良反应[J].中国药物警戒,2013,10(4):215-218.

[2] 余俭.抗菌抗病毒新药——热毒宁注射液[J].中南药学,2010,8(7):548-550.

[3] 杨红娟,李国胜,王海燕.热毒宁注射液不良反应[J].基层医学论坛,2017,21(34):4881-4882.

[4] 苗强.热毒宁注射液不良反应及预防[J].中医临床研究,2017,9(22):120-121.

[5] 康丹瑜,耿婷,丁岗,等.热毒宁注射液临床联用及药物相互作用的研究进展[J].中国药房,2017,28(2):276-279.

生脉注射液

生脉注射液是根据古方"生脉散"研制而成,临床上主要用于心肌梗死、心源性休克、感染性休克等危重症的抢救与治疗。

【主要成分】

红参、麦冬、五味子。

【药理作用及机制】

益气养阴、复脉固脱,具有心血管保护及免疫调节等功效。

1. **心血管保护作用** 生脉注射液具有抗氧化应激、抗炎作用,可提升心肌对缺氧的耐受能力,减轻心肌缺血再灌注损伤;生脉注射液可升高血浆组织型纤溶酶原水平,降低血液黏度及血浆黏度,改善组织氧代谢和血流动力学;生脉注射液对血压具有双向调节作用,即对正常患者的血压无明显影响,但使高血压患者血压降低,低血压患者血压升高;生脉注射液可提高心肌收缩力,增加心排出量,明显改善心功能。

2. 肺保护作用　生脉注射液降低动脉血二氧化碳分压、提高动脉血氧分压,改善肺功能。

3. 免疫调节作用　生脉注射液可降低血清促炎因子水平,减轻患者炎症反应,具有免疫调节功能。

【适应证】

用于心、脑血管疾病的治疗及急性胰腺炎、急性中毒、肿瘤等疾病的辅助治疗。

1. 心肌缺血、心肌梗死、心力衰竭　生脉注射液能降低血液黏度,改善老年冠心病心绞痛及心肌缺血;心肌梗死后尽早应用生脉注射液可预防病情恶化,减少并发症的发生;生脉注射液联合硝酸甘油静脉滴注治疗充血性心力衰竭,可明显增加左心室射血分数,改善心功能。

2. 肺源性心脏病　生脉注射液联合糖皮质激素静脉滴注可用于治疗肺源性心脏病,可显著降低血清酶。

3. 肿瘤化疗　生脉注射液减轻化疗药物引起的心脏毒性、肝毒性、肾毒性及急性毒性,提高患者化疗依从性。

4.《新型冠状病毒肺炎诊疗方案(试行第七版)》中,建议生脉注射液作为抗新冠肺炎治疗药物,用于新冠肺炎感染危重型患者。

【不良反应】

1. 过敏反应,如皮疹、药疹,严重者可出现过敏性休克。

2. 部分患者用药后也可出现消化系统损害,如腹胀、肝功能损害。

3. 偶发心血管系统损害,如心悸、血压下降、窦性心动过速、窦性停搏等。

【药物相互作用】

1. 本品与 0.9% 氯化钠及 10% 葡萄糖溶液配伍时,易引起溶液酸碱度变化及盐析现象,产生不溶性微粒,故建议选用 5% 葡萄糖溶液配制药物。

2. 严禁与其他药物直接混合配伍,谨慎联合用药。

3. 本品含有机酸类成分,不宜与氢氧化铝合用,以免发生中和反应,降低疗效。

4. 不宜与呋喃妥因、对氨基水杨酸、利福平、阿司匹林、苯巴比妥、苯妥英钠、吲哚美辛合用,以免提高以上药物的血药浓度,产生毒性。

5. 本品可阻碍锌的吸收,不宜同服。

6. 本品含鞣质类成分,不宜与胰酶、淀粉酶同服,以免抑制其活性,降低疗效。

7. 本品含红参,根据中药配伍禁忌,不宜与藜芦、五灵脂等药物合用。

【注意事项】

1. 本品可产生过敏等不良反应,新生儿、婴幼儿禁用;肝肾功能障碍、老年患者、生理期、孕产期女性、过敏体质患者应谨慎使用。

2. 用药过程中严格掌握适应证,做好用药监护。首次使用时,生脉注射液用量以 10~30ml 为宜,以减少不良反应发生。

3. 合并其他基础疾病患者,应在医生指导下使用。

参考文献

[1] 杨增强,敖金波,蔡兰兰,等.生脉注射液治疗急性心肌梗死后心源

性休克的临床研究[J].现代药物与临床,2017,32(1):20-24.
[2] 徐淑华,刘生友.生脉注射液的药理作用研究进展[J].中国药事,
2010,24(4):405-407.
[3] 廖名龙,郁杰,黄成斌,等.生脉注射液临床应用新进展[J].华西
药学杂志,2002,17(2):152-154.
[4] 王依蕾,袁易.生脉注射液临床应用安全性分析[J].上海医药,
2018,39(5):38-43.
[5] 涂楚.38例生脉注射液不良反应文献分析[J].海峡药学,2018,30
(4):266-268.
[6] 冯珺,曹佳薇,姚君,等.生脉注射液与常用输液配伍稳定性研究
[J].浙江中西医结合杂志,2016,26(1):82-84.

参附注射液

参附注射液来源于宋代《济生方》中的"参附汤",是"回阳救逆、益气固脱"的经典名方。

【主要成分】

红参、附片(黑顺片)。

【药理作用及机制】

回阳救逆、益气固脱,具有心血管、微循环保护及免疫调节功效。研究显示参附注射液亦具有以下已知或潜在的药理作用。

1. **抗休克作用** 参附注射液对抗内毒素引起的低血压,抑制外周动脉压持续降低;参附注射液增强右心室每搏输出量、每分输出量、射血分数和心脏指数,改善感染性休克患者的氧输送及右心室功能;参附注射液改善血液黏度,减少血小板聚集,使外周血液灌注增加,改善组织代谢,增加脑组织的血供和氧供;参附注射液保护血管内皮细胞,解除微循环血管痉挛,改善微循环。

2. **心脏保护作用** 参附注射液抑制脂质过氧化反应,降

低活性氧水平,提高心肌对缺氧的耐受力,改善受损心肌超微结构;参附注射液抑制炎症因子表达,减轻炎症反应;下调凋亡蛋白表达,减少心肌细胞凋亡,减轻缺氧损伤;增加心肌收缩力,减慢心率,降低心肌耗氧量,改善心功能,减少室性心律失常的发生。

3. 肺功能保护作用 参附注射液可抑制炎症反应,减轻内毒素引起的肺损伤;参附注射液所含的人参总皂苷和水溶性乌头碱能舒张支气管平滑肌,抑制血管痉挛,降低肺血管阻力,降低肺动脉压;参附注射液降低血液黏度和红细胞聚集性,促进纤维蛋白溶解,减少血小板聚集,加快血液流速,改善微循环,改善肺泡通气;促进肺表面活性物质合成,改善氧合。

4. 免疫调节作用 参附注射液促进细胞免疫,刺激脾淋巴细胞代谢,增强机体免疫调节及对伤害性刺激的抵抗作用;增强肝脏的解毒功能,直接对抗内毒素引起的肝、肺损伤。

〔适应证〕

参附注射液可用于阳气暴脱、气阴两亏、脉虚欲脱等证,常用于治疗休克、心力衰竭、冠心病、肺病等疾病。

1. 感染性休克 在常规西医治疗基础上联合使用参附注射液,可改善感染性休克患者微循环,显著升高患者动脉血压及中心静脉血氧饱和度;减轻脓毒血症休克患者的炎症反应,改善血流动力学;重症患者可联合应用血必净注射液。《新型冠状病毒肺炎诊疗方案(试行第七版)》中,推荐参附注射液作为抗新冠肺炎治疗药物,适用于新冠肺炎危重型患者。

2. 心肌梗死合并心力衰竭 参附注射液联合使用抗凝药物可降低心力衰竭患者炎症因子水平,改善心肌酶谱,改善心功能及患者预后。

3. 慢性阻塞性肺疾病　常规西医治疗联合参附注射液,能增加慢性阻塞性肺疾病患者血清中免疫球蛋白 IgA、IgM、IgG 的水平,增强免疫功能。

【不良反应】

1. 常见的不良反应为过敏反应,如面色潮红、烦热、口干舌燥等。

2. 偶发严重不良反应,如寒战、发热、四肢冰凉、流涎、血压及心率下降等。

【药物相互作用】

1. 本品含有红参、附片,根据中药配伍禁忌,不宜与中药半夏、瓜蒌、贝母、白蔹、白及、五灵脂、藜芦等同时使用。

2. 参附注射液与其他药物直接混合使用,可能产生不溶微粒及絮状沉淀,发生 pH 改变;若需合用,应以 0.9% 氯化钠溶液对输液管道进行冲洗。

3. 对于伴有心绞痛持续发作的患者,在使用参附注射液的基础上,宜加服硝酸酯类药物或遵医嘱。

4. 本品含黑顺片,不宜与激素类药物长期合用,以免造成患者肾阴虚,加剧体内阴精损耗。

【注意事项】

1. 本品可引起过敏等不良反应,对本品有过敏或严重不良反应病史的患者禁用。参附注射液的不良反应发生率较低,多发生于有过敏史、合并用药、超适应证、滴速过快、增大剂量、延长疗程、年老体弱者及心肺基础疾病患者,应注意加强临床用药监护,尤其是用药初始 30min 内。参附注射液引发的不良反应大多为一般不良反应,停药或对症处理后即可缓解或消失。

2. 孕妇、新生儿、婴幼儿禁用。

3. 合并其他基础疾病患者,应在医生指导下使用。

参考文献

［1］徐军,楼洪刚,楼宜嘉,等.参附注射液药理作用的研究进展［J］.上海中医药杂志,2008,42(10):87-89.

［2］曹健华.参附注射液治疗感染性休克的临床疗效分析［J］.中外医疗,2019,38(32):121-123.

［3］林翰锋.参附注射液联合血必净注射液治疗脓毒症休克对炎症指标和血流动力学的临床影响［J］.北方药学,2019,16(12):51-52.

［4］冯军鹏,梁梅芳,王有恒,等.参附注射液联合依诺肝素钠治疗急性心肌梗死并心力衰竭的疗效分析［J］.药物评价研究,2019,42(10):2057-2061.

［5］王志飞,赵维,张寅,等.基于大型前瞻性安全性监测的参附注射液不良反应影响因素分析［J］.中国中药杂志,2015,40(24):4746-4749.

参麦注射液

参麦注射液组方源于《症因脉治》中的参冬饮,具有益气固脱、养阴生津的功效,是中医理论中"扶正祛邪"的经典方剂。

【主要成分】

红参、麦冬。

【药理作用及机制】

红参补脾、益肺、益气、摄血;麦冬养阴、生津、滋阴、润燥。研究报道了参麦注射液具有以下已知及潜在的药理作用。

1. **心脏保护作用**　参麦注射液抗氧化应激损伤,稳定线粒体膜电位,减少心肌缺血缺氧后的细胞凋亡,减轻缺血损伤,改善心功能;具有膜稳定性,纠正细胞内外离子分布异常,消除缺血区心肌迟发电活动,改善冠状动脉循环与心肌代谢,预防室性心律失常;参脉注射液可激动 β 受体,抑制心肌细胞膜 Na^+-K^+-ATPase 活性,增强心肌收缩力;负性调节肾素-血管紧张素-醛固酮系统,改善心力衰竭。

2. 抗休克作用 参麦注射液可升高失血性休克动物血压;兴奋肾上腺皮质系统、促进网状内皮系统清除各种病理性物质;抑制血管平滑肌细胞膜 Na^+-K^+-ATPase 活性,促进 Ca^{2+} 内流,使外周血管收缩,增加心、肝、脑等重要脏器的血液灌注;明显提升白细胞水平,增强 IL-18 及其诱导的 γ-干扰素表达,抗多种病原微生物感染;抑制炎症反应,减轻内毒素引起的全身炎症反应综合征及多器官功能障碍综合征。

3. 免疫调节作用 减轻内毒素所致淋巴细胞凋亡;促进免疫器官发育,增强单核细胞吞噬能力,升高白细胞水平,升高血浆 γ-球蛋白、IgG、IgM 水平,增强机体非特异性免疫功能。

4. 改善肺功能 参麦注射液增加膈肌收缩力,减少膈肌细胞凋亡,改善膈肌舒张功能,降低肺动脉压及肺循环阻力,改善肺通气、肺换气;降低肺组织细胞因子水平及中性粒细胞浸润,抑制内毒素与肺泡巨噬细胞膜结合,减轻急性肺损伤。

【适应证】

用于治疗阴虚内热、气阴两虚型休克、冠心病、病毒性心肌炎、慢性肺源性心脏病。

1. 休克 常规治疗过敏性休克及创伤性休克的基础上联合应用参麦注射液,可明显提高疗效,缩短病程,迅速升高血压,控制病情进展。

2. 肺源性心脏病 参麦注射液可改善肺源性心脏病患者左心室收缩功能,改善慢性肺源性心脏病患者血液黏度及缺氧症状,可缩短病程,减少呼吸衰竭的发生。

3. 心肌缺血及心力衰竭　参麦注射液可用于预防急性心肌缺血 - 再灌注损伤,减少心肌耗氧量,缩小梗死面积,改善左心室射血分数,提高治疗有效率,降低出血及再灌注心律失常等并发症的发生率;有效治疗充血性心力衰竭,改善心力衰竭患者临床体征及心功能,改善血流动力学及微循环。

4.《新型冠状病毒肺炎诊疗方案(试行第七版)》推荐参麦注射液作为抗新冠肺炎治疗药物,适用于新冠肺炎危重症伴有免疫抑制的患者。

【不良反应】

参麦注射液可引起过敏反应,如呼吸困难、气喘、颜面青紫、四肢发凉、口周流涎,严重者可出现过敏性休克。部分患者使用后,亦可出现皮肤损害及消化系统损害,如皮疹、剥脱性皮炎、腹痛、腹胀等,循环系统症状,如心动过速及低血压等,停药后症状可消失或缓解。

【药物相互作用】

1. 参麦注射液不宜与藜芦、五灵脂及其制剂配伍使用。

2. 参麦注射液不宜与甘油果糖注射液、青霉素类高敏类药物联合使用。

【注意事项】

1. 本品可引起过敏等不良反应,对含有红参、麦冬制剂过敏或有严重不良反应史的患者禁用。

2. 新生儿、婴幼儿、孕妇、哺乳期妇女禁用;肝、肾功能异常患者,老年患者慎用。

3. 本品可引起心动过速及低血压等症状,有心脏严重疾病患者慎用。

4. 本品中含有的红参可提高机体兴奋性,不宜与强心苷类药物、中枢兴奋药物同用,以免发生中毒。

5. 合并其他基础疾病患者,应在医生指导下使用。

参考文献

［1］尹丽慧,沃兴德.参麦注射液的药理和临床研究进展[J].浙江中医学院学报,2011,25(6):65-68.

［2］曹旭东,丁志山,陈建.参麦注射液药理及临床研究进展[J].中国中医药信息杂志,2010,17(3):104-106.

［3］吴青业,刘冬梅.参麦注射液的临床应用[J].中国医院药学杂志,2000,20(11):676-678.

［4］刘蔚红,李成建,张筠,等.参麦注射液不良反应[J].中国误诊学杂志,2011,11(31):7690.

［5］闫正博.浅析参麦注射液联合应用及不良反应[J].药物与临床,2019,19(91):132-133.

清肺排毒汤

清肺排毒汤是针对此次新型冠状病毒肺炎研制的创新特效方剂。其组方来源于张仲景《伤寒论》中经典方剂麻杏石甘汤、射干麻黄汤、小柴胡汤、五苓散等的优化组合。目前在山西、河北、黑龙江、陕西四省试点医院使用,反馈良好。

【推荐处方】

麻黄 9g、炙甘草 6g、杏仁 9g、生石膏 15~30g(先煎)、桂枝 9g、泽泻 9g、猪苓 9g、白术 9g、茯苓 15g、柴胡 16g、黄芩 6g、姜半夏 9g、生姜 9g、紫菀 9g、冬花 9g、射干 9g、细辛 6g、山药 12g、枳实 6g、陈皮 6g、藿香 9g。

【药理作用及机制】

麻杏石甘汤具有解表作用,有辛凉宣泄、清肺平喘的功效。射干麻黄汤具有宣肺祛痰,下气止咳之功效,适用于新冠肺炎憋闷气短、咳嗽等症状。五苓散方为医圣张仲景所创,功用化气利水。现代药理研究表明小柴胡汤具有退热、抗炎、免疫调节、镇吐、保肝、利胆等方面的作用。加之藿香芳香化湿,石膏防郁化热,优化组合后的方剂可宣肺止咳,祛寒除湿,保肝利胆。

【适应证】

清肺排毒汤在《新型冠状病毒肺炎诊疗方案(试行第七版)》推荐为确诊病例的临床治疗期用药。适用范围:适用于轻型、普通型、重型患者,在危重型患者救治中可结合患者实际情况合理使用。

【用法用量】

《新型冠状病毒肺炎诊疗方案(试行第七版)》推荐清肺排毒汤服用方法为:

1. 传统中药饮片,水煎服。每日一付,早晚两次(饭后40min),温服,三付一个疗程。

2. 如有条件,每次服完药可加服大米汤半碗,舌干津液亏虚者可多服至一碗(米汤可清胃部虚热,保护胃气,早在《本草纲目拾遗》中便有记载,具有滋阴的功效)。

【注意事项】

1. 如患者不发热则生石膏的用量要小,发热或壮热可加大生石膏用量(生石膏肺热咳喘有效,为大寒之物,容易伤阳气,过量使用会出现胃口欠佳,精神不振,浑身无力等情况)。生石膏有清热泻火的作用,风寒感冒者禁用,孕妇慎用,儿童、哺乳期妇女、年老体弱及脾虚便溏者应在医师指导下服用。

2. 按照《新型冠状病毒肺炎诊疗方案(试行第七版)》推荐,若症状好转而未痊愈则服用第2个疗程,若患者有特殊情况或其他基础病,第2个疗程可以根据实际情况修改处方,症状消失则停药。

3. 根据新冠肺炎确诊病例使用该方剂时的报道,依据个体差异,在个体用药中有可能需要微调剂量,请在医师的指导下使用。

4. 本品中含有麻黄,使用麻黄时易发汗过多而损气,不宜剂量过大或者长期服用。麻黄与生物碱类药物同用可使毒性增加,与强心苷类药物同用增加强心苷毒性,诱发心律失常。

5. 本品中含有黄芩成分,对本品成分有过敏史者禁用,过敏体质者慎用。

6. 服用本品期间,若服用其他药物应先咨询医师。

参考文献

[1] 姜雪,孙森凤,王悦.麻黄的毒性作用研究概况[J].山东化工,2017,46(14):49-50,54.

[2] 余永鑫,唐文,王建挺.五苓散经方新用的临证思路探讨[J].中医药通报,2019,18(06):22-24.

[3] 孙明瑜.小柴胡汤配伍与药理作用相关性的研究[D].北京:北京中医药大学,2003.

寒湿郁肺证方剂

【推荐处方】

生麻黄 6g、生石膏 15g、杏仁 9g、羌活 15g、葶苈子 15g、贯众 9g、地龙 15g、徐长卿 15g、藿香 15g、佩兰 9g、苍术 15g、云苓 45g、生白术 30g、焦三仙各 9g、厚朴 15g、焦槟榔 9g、煨草果 9g、生姜 15g。

【药理作用及机制】

麻黄主要成分为麻黄碱,具有缓解支气管平滑肌痉挛、利尿、抗炎、抗病毒作用。麻黄、生姜合用加强排汗、止咳、祛痰作用;麻黄、杏仁合用具有止咳平喘功效;麻黄、白术、石膏合用清肺平喘;厚朴含各种酚类物质,其中厚朴酚为主要成分之一,其主要作用有抗菌、抗炎及肌肉松弛;苍术含有多种挥发油,油中主含苍术醇,具有镇静、松弛平滑肌作用;佩兰含有聚伞花素,具有抗菌、抗病毒以及祛痰作用;佩兰、苍术、厚朴合用可治湿阻中焦之证。

藿香含有挥发油,油中主要成分为广藿香醇,增强消化能力,收敛止泻,发汗;槟榔、厚朴、草果合用治疗湿热中阻,枢纽失职;苍术、焦三仙合用燥湿运脾,行气和胃;草果含有蒎烯,具有镇咳祛痰、抗炎、抗菌、促消化、利尿作用,与云苓、葶苈子合用,增强利尿作用。

地龙含有多种氨基酸,具有清热解毒、平喘止咳作用,与麻黄、杏仁合用,加强清肺化痰、止咳平喘之功效,与羌活、贯众合用增强其解热镇痛、抗病毒之功效;徐长卿主含丹皮酚、黄酮苷和少量生物碱,具有镇痛、镇静、抗菌、降压、降血脂等多种作用。

【适应证】

发热,乏力,周身酸痛,咳嗽,咯痰,胸紧憋气,纳呆,恶心,呕吐,大便黏腻不爽;舌质淡伴有齿痕或淡红,苔白厚腐腻或白腻,脉濡或滑。《新型冠状毒肺炎诊疗方案(试行第七版)》推荐有以上临床表现轻症患者服用此方剂。

【用法用量】

《新型冠状病毒肺炎诊疗方案(试行第七版)》建议每日1剂,水煎600ml,分3次服用,早、中、晚各1次,饭前服用。

【注意事项】

该方多为辛苦温燥湿之药物,易耗气伤津,故气虚津亏者、体弱者、孕妇慎用;贯众切忌油腻,脂肪可引起贯众毒性反应,引起头痛、腹泻等症状;生白术便秘者切忌服用;患者使用该方务必饮食忌生冷、油腻与辛辣之物。

湿热蕴肺证方剂

【推荐处方】

槟榔 10g、草果 10g、厚朴 10g、知母 10g、黄芩 10g、柴胡 10g、赤芍 10g、连翘 15g、青蒿 10g(后下)、苍术 10g、大青叶 10g、生甘草 5g。

【药理作用及机制】

连翘含三萜皂苷,具有广谱抗菌、抗病毒、解热、降血压等作用;甘草含有三萜类成分,具有祛痰平喘、抗菌、抗病毒、抗炎等作用,与连翘合用,增强清热解毒之功效;黄芩含有黄芩苷元,具有解热、降压、镇静、抗菌、抗病毒等作用;柴胡含有柴胡皂苷以及多种挥发油成分,具有镇静、镇痛、解热、镇咳等广泛中枢抑制作用,与黄芩同用,增强清热解表、治疗发热头痛作用;青蒿含有倍半萜类、黄酮类、香豆素类等成分,具有抗疟疾、解热镇痛、抗菌、抗病毒之功效,与黄芩合用增强其抗病毒、解热镇痛之功效;苍术含有多种挥发油,油中主含苍术醇,对中枢神经系统具有镇静作用,松弛平滑肌。

草果含有蒎烯,具有镇咳祛痰、抗炎、抗菌、促进消化、利尿作用。槟榔含有槟榔碱,主要有驱虫、抗病毒、促进消化等作用,与草果同用可以增强抗菌、抗病毒、驱虫之功效。

厚朴含有厚朴酚,具有抗菌、抗炎、中枢性肌肉松弛作用;赤芍含有芍药苷等成分,具有镇静、抗炎止痛、解热、抗惊厥之功效,与黄芩合用增强其清热解毒之功效;大青叶主含多种氨基酸、靛玉红 B 等成分,具有抗菌、抗病毒、清热解毒作用;知母含有知母皂苷等成分,具有解热、抗菌、抗病毒作用。

【适应证】

低热或不发热,微恶寒,乏力,头身困重,肌肉酸痛,干咳痰少,咽痛,口干不欲多饮,或伴有胸闷脘痞,无汗或汗出不畅,或见呕恶纳呆,便溏或大便黏滞不爽。舌淡红,苔白厚腻或薄黄,脉滑数或濡数。《新型冠状病毒肺炎诊疗方案(试行第七版)》推荐有以上临床表现轻症患者服用此方剂。

【用法用量】

《新型冠状病毒肺炎诊疗方案(试行第七版)》建议每日1剂,水煎400ml,分2次服用,早晚各1次。

【注意事项】

该方多为苦寒、清热解表之药物,易伤胃伤脾,故脾胃虚寒者、体弱者、孕妇慎用;甘草切忌与京大戟、芫花、甘遂、海藻同用;赤芍反藜芦,不能同用;患者使用该方务必饮食忌生冷、油腻与辛辣之物。

参考文献

[1] 苗磊,亓超.麻黄杏仁甘草石膏汤证浅述[J].菏泽医学专科学校学报,2011,23(04):46-47.
[2] 胡方媛,范玉浩,范欣生,等.厚朴麻黄汤对哮喘小鼠气道炎症及TRPA1、TRPV1 mRNA与蛋白表达的影响[J].中国实验方剂学杂志,2020,26(01):37-42.
[3] 王东梅,王莹莹,穆云婧,等.茯苓杏仁甘草汤治疗雾霾吸入性肺损伤的可行性分析[J].河北中医,2019,41(05):771-774.
[4] 蒋伟,薛琴,李洁,等.麻黄连翘赤豆汤加减治疗湿热咳嗽的临床效果[J].解放军医药杂志,2019,31(10):85-88.

湿毒郁肺证方剂

【推荐处方】

生麻黄6g、苦杏仁15g、生石膏30g、生薏苡仁30g、茅苍术10g、广藿香15g、青蒿草12g、虎杖20g、马鞭草30g、干芦根30g、葶苈子15g、化橘红15g、生甘草10g。

【药理作用及机制】

生麻黄主要活性成分为麻黄碱、阿魏酰组胺等,具有镇痛、抗菌、抗病毒、抗炎、解热、降压、利尿、平喘作用;苦杏仁主要活性成分为苦杏仁苷、脂肪油、苦杏仁酶等,具有镇咳平喘、抗炎镇痛、抗氧化、润肠通便、降血脂、调节免疫功能的作用;生石膏具有解热、镇痛、提高免疫力的作用。

生薏苡仁主要活性成分为薏苡仁酯、脂肪酸,具有降脂、抗炎镇痛、提高免疫力的作用;茅苍术主要活性成分为苍术素、茅术醇,具有缓解肠道痉挛、保护胃黏膜、抗菌的作用;广藿香主要活性成分为广藿香酮、β-丁香烯等,具有抗病毒、抗菌、抗真菌、促消化、抗炎镇痛和解热作用;青蒿草主要活性成分为青蒿素,具有抗疟、抗菌、抗病毒、抗心律失常作用。

虎杖主要活性成分为蒽醌类化合物,具有抗菌、镇咳平喘、降压、抗病毒、抗肿瘤、镇静、改善微循环作用;马鞭草主要活性成分为马鞭草苷,具有抗炎止痛、镇咳、抗疟、抗菌作用;干芦根主要化学成分为多糖类,具有保肝、抗菌作用;葶苈子主要活性成分为芥子苷,具有止咳平喘、强心、抗菌作用;化橘红主要活性成分为柠檬醛,具有镇静、抗微生物、止咳化痰作用;生甘草主要活性成分为甘草苷,具有抗菌、抗病毒、抗炎、镇咳解痉、抗过敏作用。

【适应证】

该方剂主治湿毒郁肺证,《新型冠状病毒肺炎诊疗方案(试行第七版)》中推荐普通型新冠肺炎患者使用。临床表现为:发热,咳嗽痰少,或有黄痰,憋闷气促,腹胀,便秘不畅,舌质暗红,舌体胖,苔黄腻或黄燥,脉滑数或弦滑。

【用法用量】

《新型冠状病毒肺炎诊疗方案(试行第七版)》建议每日1剂,水煎400ml,分2次服用,早晚各1次。

【注意事项】

1. 该方剂含有生麻黄,体虚自汗、盗汗及虚喘者禁服。

2. 该方剂中含有生薏苡仁,脾约便难者及孕妇慎用,胃虚者慎用。

3. 该方剂中含有青蒿草,产后血虚,内寒作泻及饮食停滞泄泻者不可使用。

4. 该方剂中含有甘草,有中枢神经抑制作用,故婴幼儿及老年患者不宜大量长期服用;此外,甘草有升高血压的作用,高血压患者不宜大量长期服用,急性肾炎患者忌用,醛固酮增多症、低钾血症患者禁用。

寒湿阻肺证方剂

【推荐处方】

苍术 15g、陈皮 10g、厚朴 10g、藿香 10g、草果 6g、生麻黄 6g、羌活 10g、生姜 10g、槟榔 10g。

【药理作用及机制】

苍术主要活性成分为苍术醇、茅术醇、β- 桉叶醇等,对结核分枝杆菌、金黄色葡萄球菌、大肠埃希菌及铜绿假单胞菌有显著抑制效果,同时具有抗炎、促进消化吸收和免疫调节作用;陈皮具有保护心脏、祛痰平喘、消胀止呕等药理作用;厚朴煎剂对肺炎球菌、白喉杆菌、溶血性链球菌、金黄色葡萄球菌及多种皮肤真菌均有抑制作用。

藿香挥发油能促进胃液分泌,增强消化能力,对胃肠有解痉作用,同时具备抗菌、止泻、扩张微血管等作用;草果的主要活性成分为 1,8- 桉叶素,具有镇咳祛痰、镇痛、解热、平喘、抗菌、抗炎作用;生麻黄主要活性成分为麻黄碱,具有镇痛、抗菌、抗病毒、抗炎、解热、降压、利尿、平喘作用;羌活主要活性成分为香豆素类化合物,具有解热、镇痛、抗炎、抗心律失常作用。

生姜主要活性成分为姜醇、姜烯等,对金黄色葡萄球菌、表皮葡萄球菌、伤寒杆菌、宋内痢疾杆菌、铜绿假单胞菌均有明显抑制作用,此外还具有抗血小板聚集、兴奋呼吸系统、镇静、抗氧化作用;槟榔具有促进消化吸收、抗病原微生物作用。

【适应证】

该方剂主治寒湿阻肺证,《新型冠状病毒肺炎诊疗方案(试行第七版)》推荐普通型新冠肺炎患者使用。临床表现为:低热,身热不扬,或未热,干咳,少痰,倦怠乏力,胸闷,脘痞,或呕恶,便溏,舌质淡或淡红,苔白或白腻,脉濡。

【用法用量】

《新型冠状病毒肺炎诊疗方案(试行第七版)》建议每日 1 剂,水煎 400ml,分 2 次服用,早晚各 1 次。

【注意事项】

1. 该方剂含有苍术,阴虚内热,气虚多汗者不可使用。

2. 该方剂含有厚朴,孕妇不宜使用。

3. 该方剂含有生麻黄,体虚自汗、盗汗及虚喘者禁服。

参考文献

张明发,沈雅琴. 中药苍术炮制前后药理作用的研究进展[J]. 抗感染药学,2017,14(03):481-485.

疫毒闭肺证方剂

【推荐处方】

生麻黄 6g、杏仁 9g、生石膏 15g、甘草 3g、藿香 10g(后下)、厚朴 10g、苍术 15g、草果 10g、法半夏 9g、茯苓 15g、生大黄 5g(后下)、生黄芪 10g、葶苈子 10g、赤芍 10g。

【药理作用及机制】

生麻黄主要活性成分为麻黄碱,具有镇痛、抗菌、抗病毒、抗炎、解热、降压、利尿、平喘作用;杏仁主要活性成分为苦杏仁苷、脂肪油、苦杏仁酶等,具有镇咳平喘、抗炎镇痛、抗氧化、润肠通便、降血脂、调节免疫功能的作用;生石膏具有解热、镇痛、提高免疫力的作用。

甘草主要活性成分为甘草苷,具有抗菌、抗病毒、抗炎、镇咳解痉、抗过敏作用;藿香挥发油能促进胃液分泌,增强消化能力,对胃肠有解痉作用,同时具备抗菌、止泻、扩张微血管等作用;厚朴煎剂对肺炎球菌、白喉杆菌、溶血性链球菌、金黄色葡萄球菌及多种皮肤真菌均有抑制作用;苍术主要活性成分为苍术素、茅术醇等,具有缓解肠道痉挛、保护胃黏膜、抗菌作用;草果主要活性成分1,8-桉叶素,具有镇咳祛痰、镇痛、解热、平喘、抗菌、抗炎作用。

法半夏为半夏的炮制加工品,主要活性成分为3-乙酰氨基-5-甲基异噁唑等,具有镇咳、止吐、抗心律失常、降压、促凝血作用;茯苓主要活性成分为β-茯苓聚糖,具有利尿、抗菌作用;生大黄主要活性成分为大黄酸、大黄素、芦荟大黄素等,具有促消化、抗菌、降脂、缓解支气管痉挛、促进血液凝固的作用;生黄芪主要活性成分为黄芪苷,具有提高免疫力、抗菌、抗病毒、利尿作用;葶苈子主要活性成分为芥子苷,具有止咳平喘、强心、抗菌作用;赤芍主要活性成分为芍药苷,具有抗血小板聚集、抗血栓形成、保肝作用。

【适应证】

该方剂主治疫毒闭肺证,《新型冠状病毒肺炎诊疗方案(试行第七版)》推荐重型新冠肺炎患者使用。临床表现为:发热面红,咳嗽,痰黄黏少,或痰中带血,喘憋气促,疲乏倦怠,口干苦黏,恶心不食,大便不畅,小便短赤,舌红,苔黄腻,脉滑数。

【用法用量】

《新型冠状病毒肺炎诊疗方案(试行第七版)》建议每日 1~2 剂,水煎服,每次 100~200ml,1 日 2~4 次,口服或鼻饲。

【注意事项】

1. 该方剂含有生麻黄,体虚自汗、盗汗及虚喘者禁服。

2. 该方剂含有厚朴,孕妇不宜使用。

3. 该方剂含有法半夏,不宜与乌头类药物合用,一切血证及阴虚燥咳、津伤口渴者忌服。

气营两燔证方剂

【推荐处方】

生石膏 30~60g(先煎)、知母 30g、生地 30~60g、水牛角 30g(先煎)、赤芍 30g、玄参 30g、连翘 15g、丹皮 15g、黄连 6g、竹叶 12g、葶苈子 15g、生甘草 6g。

【药理作用及机制】

生石膏具有解热、镇痛、提高免疫力的作用;知母主要活性成分为知母皂苷及其他皂苷元,具有抗菌和促肾上腺皮质激素分泌的作用;生地水提液具有抗肺纤维化、促进造血、抗炎、改善糖脂代谢、保护胃黏膜的功能。

水牛角主要活性成分为胆甾醇及各种氨基酸,具有强心、镇静、抗惊厥作用;赤芍主要活性成分为芍药苷,具有抗血小板聚集、抗血栓形成、保肝作用;玄参具有抗细菌、抗真菌、镇静、降压、强心、扩张血管、抗惊厥作用;连翘主要活性成分为连翘酚和连翘苷,具有抗菌、止吐、强心、利尿作用;丹皮主要活性成分为牡丹酚,具有抗菌、镇静、催眠、镇痛、降压作用。

黄连主要成分为小檗碱,具有抗菌、抗心律失常、止泻、抗炎作用;竹叶主要活性成分为竹叶多糖和黄酮类,具有抗氧化、抗心肌缺血、收缩血管、抑菌和肝损伤保护等作用;葶苈子主要活性成分为芥子苷,具有止咳平喘、强心、抗菌作用;生甘草主要活性成分为甘草苷,具有抗菌、抗病毒、抗炎、镇咳解痉、抗过敏作用。

【适应证】

该方剂主治气营两燔证,《新型冠状病毒肺炎诊疗方案(试行第七版)》中推荐重型新冠肺炎患者使用。临床表现为:大热烦渴,喘憋气促,谵语神昏,视物错瞀,或发斑疹,或吐血、衄血,或四肢抽搐,舌绛少苔或无苔,脉沉细数,或浮大而数。

【用法用量】

《新型冠状病毒肺炎诊疗方案(试行第七版)》建议每日 1 剂,水煎服,先煎石膏、水牛角后下诸药,每次 100~200ml,每日 2~4 次,口服或鼻饲。

【注意事项】

1. 该方剂含有水牛角,中虚胃寒者慎服,大量服用后常有上腹部不适、恶心、腹胀、食欲缺乏等反应。

2. 该方剂含有赤芍,血虚无瘀之症及痈疽已溃者慎服。

3. 该方剂含有玄参,不宜与藜芦同用,脾胃有湿及脾虚便溏者忌服。

4. 该方剂含有连翘,脾胃虚弱,气虚发热,痈疽已溃、脓稀色淡者忌服。

5. 该方剂含有丹皮,血虚有寒,孕妇及月经过多者慎服。

6. 该方剂含有黄连,黄连性大寒,过量久服易伤脾胃,脾胃虚寒者忌用,此外,黄连苦燥易伤阴津,阴虚津伤者慎用。

7. 该方剂中含有甘草,甘草有抗惊厥等中枢神经抑制作用,故婴幼儿及老年患者不宜大量长期服用;此外,甘草有升高血压的作用,高血压患者不宜大量长期服用,急性肾炎患者忌用,醛固酮增多症、低钾血症患者禁用。

参考文献

梁丹,陈奇兰,陈清霞.竹叶药理作用研究进展[J].临床合理用药杂志,2014,7(11):89-90.

内闭外脱证方剂

【推荐处方】

人参 15g、黑顺片 10g(先煎)、山茱萸 15g,送服苏合香丸或安宫牛黄丸。

1. 安宫牛黄丸成分为　牛黄、水牛角浓缩粉、人工麝香、珍珠、朱砂、雄黄、黄连、黄芩、栀子、郁金、冰片。

2. 苏合香丸成分为　苏合香、安息香、冰片、水牛角浓缩粉、人工麝香、檀香、沉香、丁香、香附、木香、乳香(制)、荜茇、白术、诃子肉、朱砂。

【药理作用及机制】

人参复脉固脱、生津安神;黑顺片补脾助阳、散寒止痛,与人参同为"回阳救逆"之良药;山茱萸生津止渴、涩精固脱;合用药物安宫牛黄丸源自清代吴瑭的《温病条辨》,是传统中药中的经典急救方,与紫雪丹、至宝丹一起,被誉为"中医温病凉开三宝",可清热解毒,镇惊开窍;苏合香丸是著名的温通开窍药,可芳香开窍,行气止痛。

研究表明,人参中主要成分人参皂苷具有抗炎、抗氧化、抗衰老、心血管保护等多种作用;黑顺片中主要成分乌头碱具有明显的强心、抗炎、镇痛等功效;山茱萸中所含的多糖、有机酸及环烯醚萜类物质也具有抗炎、镇痛、强心、调节内分泌等功效。

合用药安宫牛黄丸组方中黄连、黄芩中含有的小檗碱和黄芩苷具有清热泻火的功效,能明显对抗细菌毒素引起的发热;牛黄、朱砂抑制中枢神经系统兴奋性,起镇静、催眠、抗惊厥作用;麝香含有的麝香酮可改善中枢神经系统功能、减轻脑缺血缺氧损伤;冰片含右旋龙脑,对大肠埃希菌、金黄色葡萄球菌有抑制作用;珍珠、牛黄合用可抑制真菌感染。

合用药苏合香丸具有抗炎、心血管保护、神经功能保护等多种药理作用。主要成分苏合香具有抑制血小板聚集、抗心肌缺血、抑制血管收缩、抗氧化等作用,可减轻心肌缺血损伤,保护心肌细胞;苏合香含有的脂溶挥发性成分使其能透过血脑屏障,减轻神经细胞自由基损伤及炎症反应,保护缺血缺氧损伤的神经细胞,减轻脑缺血再灌注损伤;苏合香有效成分桂皮酸具有抑菌、防腐、止泻及升高白细胞的作用,可缓解局部炎症。

【适应证】

人参、黑顺片、山茱萸合用,可治疗肺虚喘咳、气短喘促、亡阳虚脱、肢冷脉微等气血津液不足之证;合用安宫牛黄丸,可用于脑炎、脑膜炎、中毒性脑病、脑出血、败血症、脑卒中引起的高热惊厥、神昏谵语;合用苏合香丸,可用于痰迷心窍所致的痰厥昏迷、中风偏瘫、惊痫等。该处方可用于上呼吸道感染、肺炎、急性扁桃体炎、急性肠炎等引起的发热,有效改善喘憋状态及腹胀症状;也可用于病毒性脑炎引起的发热、头痛、抽搐、意识障碍;配合西药使用可治疗以"痰浊蒙心"为主证的肺性脑病;辅助治疗急性重型颅脑损伤、脑动脉硬化症、脑卒中及心绞痛。《新型冠状病毒肺炎诊疗方案(试行第七版)》推荐此方用于新冠肺炎危重症患者内闭外脱证,可减轻患者呼吸困难、气喘、神昏烦躁、汗出肢冷等症状。

【用法用量】

《新型冠状病毒肺炎诊疗方案(试行第七版)》建议使用该处方治疗新型冠状病毒感染的危重型患者,用法为:人参15g、黑顺片 10g（先煎）、山茱萸 15g，送服苏合香丸或安宫牛黄丸。安宫牛黄丸及苏合香丸均为中成药，不同剂型及制药厂家不同，建议参考药品说明书服用，切勿过量使用。

【注意事项】

1. 单次大量使用该处方的患者易发生过敏反应，主要表现为皮疹、荨麻疹，严重者可引起过敏性休克。

2. 处方中安宫牛黄丸易引起呼吸困难、恶心、呕吐、腹泻等症状。

3. 处方中安宫牛黄丸含有雄黄，其主要成分为硫化砷，长期服用可出现砷中毒，表现为皮肤损伤，如皮肤干燥、丘疹、疱疹、剥脱性皮炎、色素沉着等。不宜与亚硝酸盐类、亚铁盐类、硝酸盐、硫酸盐类药物合用，避免疗效下降或增加毒性；不宜与酶类药物同用，以免形成不溶性沉淀而抑制酶活性。

4. 处方中安宫牛黄丸及苏合香丸中均含有朱砂，其主要成分为硫化汞，长期服用可引起神经毒性、肝肾毒性、生殖毒性，急性中毒时可出现昏迷甚至死亡。

5. 处方中人参可提高机体兴奋性，不宜与强心苷类药物、中枢兴奋药物同用，以免发生中毒；人参皂苷在酸性环境中易水解失效，不宜与酸性较强的药物合用；人参皂苷与含金属的盐类药物易形成沉淀，不宜同服。

6. 处方中含人参、黑顺片，黑顺片即为附子的炮制品之一，根据中药配伍禁忌，该方不宜与藜芦、五灵脂、半夏、瓜蒌、贝母、白蔹、白及等药物同用。

7. 该处方不宜与激素类药物长期合用，以免造成患者肾阴虚，加剧体内阴精损耗。

8. 该处方不宜与小檗碱同服，以免处方中氨基酸类物质影响小檗碱的抗菌作用。

9. 该方药性猛烈，服用时应严格掌握用量和服用时间，不可过量服用。

10. 肝肾功能异常者、老年人、儿童、孕妇不宜服用该处方,以免中毒。

11. 合并其他基础疾病患者,应在医生指导下服用。

参考文献

［1］李丹,李秀明,周宁.安宫牛黄丸的药理作用及临床新应用[J].海军医学杂志,2007,28(2):179-181.

［2］王洋,徐珠屏,王建,等.苏合香概述[J].中药与临床,2013,4(3):49-51.

［3］边晶,张洪义.苏合香古今应用初探[J].中医药临床杂志,2016,28(6):875-878.

［4］陈路遥,佘蓉,马佳燕,等.雄黄的临床不良反应分析[J].中医药信息,2018,35(6):17-20.

［5］丁通,骆骄阳,韩旭,等.朱砂毒性的研究进展及配伍必要性分析[J].中国中药杂志,2016,41(24):4533-4540.

［6］单梅,魏风菊.朱砂与含溴化物类药物的配伍禁忌[J].河北职工医学院学报,2001,18(1):46.

［7］康杰尧,李世杰,王艳,等.东北刺人参化学成分及药理作用研究进展[J].中成药,2020,42(1):156-161.

［8］袁雯.附子的药理研究[J].中医临床研究,2018,10(4):145-147.

［9］周迎春,张廉洁,张燕丽.山茱萸化学成分及药理作用研究新进展[J].中医药信息,2020,37(1):114-120.

肺脾气虚证方剂

【推荐处方】

法半夏 9g、陈皮 10g、党参 15g、炙黄芪 30g、炒白术 10g、茯苓 15g、藿香 10g、砂仁 6g(后下)、甘草 6g。

【药理作用及机制】

此方为六君子汤剂的修订版,六君子汤主要由人参、白术、茯苓、甘草、陈皮、半夏等药物组合而成,具有益气健脾、燥湿化痰之效,其中半夏、陈皮具有燥湿化痰、平喘止呕之效;白术、人参具有补气健脾、燥湿利水之效;茯苓、甘草具有益气和中、调脾化湿化痰之效。上述药物协同,使该方剂具有减少炎症细胞浸润,抑制胃酸分泌与胃黏膜病变,调节免疫功能的作用。

此处方中增加了炙黄芪、藿香与砂仁。黄芪具有补气升阳、利尿脱毒、固表止汗之效,可增强免疫力、降低血压、保护心血管、调节血糖、抑制病毒等;藿香可调节胃肠道功能,具有抗菌、抗病毒、抗炎、镇痛解热等作用;砂仁可化湿止呕、降气咳痰、解酒醒神,具有增进肠道蠕动、抑制血小板聚集等作用。

【适应证】

该方剂适用于气短,倦怠乏力,纳差呕恶,痞满,大便无力,便溏不爽,舌淡胖,苔白腻患者。《新型冠状病毒肺炎诊疗方案(试行第七版)》推荐恢复期患者使用该方剂。

【用法用量】

《新型冠状病毒肺炎诊疗方案(试行第七版)》中建议每日1剂,水煎400ml,分2次服用,早晚各1次。

【注意事项】

1. 患者服用此方剂时饮食应注意忌食生冷、油腻与辛辣之物。

2. 法半夏可降低乌头类抗炎活性,不宜与乌头类药材同用。

3. 黄芪具有助热补火之效,湿热或易过敏患者禁用。

4. 砂仁易引起过敏反应,表现为腹部与生殖器出现皮疹或团块,若出现过敏反应应立即停药。

参考文献

[1] 孙亮,戴逸飞,陆雪秋,等.基于系统药理方法挖掘六君子汤的关键

靶点与治疗疾病[J].环球中医药,2018,11(02):62-68.

[2] 张国用.中药黄芪的药理作用及其临床应用研究[J].实用心脑肺血管病杂志,2012,20(06):135-136.

[3] 任守忠,靳德军,张俊清,等.广藿香药理作用研究进展[J].中国现代中药,2006,8(8):27-29.

[4] 柯斌,师林.砂仁临床功效探究[J].中华中医药杂志,2012,27(01):132-133.

[5] 赖珍珍,张凌,李莹,等."半夏反草乌"减弱抗炎效应及其减效机制[J].中国实验方剂学杂志,2015,21(17):84-87.

气阴两虚证方剂

【推荐处方】

南北沙参各 10g、麦冬 15g、西洋参 6g,五味子 6g、生石膏 15g、淡竹叶 10g、桑叶 10g、芦根 15g、丹参 15g、生甘草 6g。

【药理作用及机制】

此方为竹叶石膏汤增减后的处方。竹叶石膏汤具有清热生津,益气和胃之效。淡竹叶富含黄酮、多糖类成分,可清除体内自由基,具有抗菌、抗肿瘤、抗衰老等作用;生石膏与麦冬可调节巨噬细胞和网状细胞内皮系统功能;甘草具有抗炎、抗氧化、抗肿瘤等作用。

此处方中增加了西洋参,南北沙参,五味子,桑叶,芦根,丹参。西洋参具有抗疲劳、抗缺氧、抗肿瘤、保护心血管、降低血小板聚集、调节细胞免疫、保护肝脏损伤等作用;南北沙参均具有镇咳祛痰的药理作用,在治疗呼吸系统疾病时可联合应用,北沙参还具有解热镇痛、增强免疫力的作用;五味子对中枢神经系统、肝脏、免疫功能、心血管系统均具有保护作用,此外五味子可兴奋呼吸系统,加深加快呼吸;桑叶亦可治疗咳嗽,明目止渴,降压调脂;芦根具有保肝、抗菌、抗炎等作用,对支气管炎、急性扁桃体炎、感冒等效果显著;丹参的主要成分为丹参酮,具有显著的抗菌消炎、活血祛瘀、心肌保护、抗肿瘤作用。

【适应证】

《新型冠状病毒肺炎诊疗方案(试行第七版)》推荐恢复期患者使用该方剂,该方剂适用于乏力,气短,口干,口渴,心悸,汗多,纳差,低热或不热,干咳少痰,舌干少津,脉细或虚无力的患者。

【用法用量】

《新型冠状病毒肺炎诊疗方案(试行第七版)》建议每日1剂,水煎 400ml,分 2 次服用,早晚各 1 次。

【注意事项】

1. 西洋参会导致过敏反应,加剧心律失常、女性内分泌紊乱等不良反应。

2. 五味子可致部分患者胃酸分泌增多或胃痛,不建议长期服用。

3. 北沙参可致过敏性皮炎。

4. 竹叶石膏汤清凉质润,痰湿或阳虚发热患者忌用。

5. 竹叶性寒,脾胃虚寒者禁用。

参考文献

[1] 路军章,张昭,赵红,等.竹叶石膏汤的核心脉证及主治疾病研究[J].中华中医药杂志,2011,26(12):58-60.

[2] 舒思洁.西洋参及其活性成分的药理学研究进展[J].时珍国医国药,2006,17(12):2603-2604.

[3] 陈文华.南、北沙参的现代药理作用比较[J].中外健康文摘:医药月刊,2008,5(4):251-253.

[4] 郭冷秋,张鹏,黄莉莉,等.五味子药理作用研究进展[J].中医药学报,2006,34(4):51-53.

[5] 孙淑玲.中药芦根的药理作用及临床应用[J].中西医结合心血管病电子杂志,2016,4(36):165.

Antiviral drugs

Arbidol

Arbidol is a non-nucleoside and broad-spectrum antiviral drug.

Pharmacokinetics

Arbidol is rapidly absorbed orally. The blood concentration reaches a peak 1.38h after administration, and the plasma protein binding rate is as high as 90%. Arbidol is metabolized with a $t_{1/2}$ of 15.7h by the liver and excreted from bile. It is widely distributed in the body with the highest enrichment in the liver.

Pharmacologic Effects and Mechanism

Arbidol is a broad-spectrum antiviral drug that blocks virus replication by inhibiting virus invasion through fusion of lipid membranes with host cells. A large number of studies have shown that arbidol exerts inhibitory effects on various viruses such as influenza A virus, influenza B virus, respiratory syncytial virus, Coxsackie virus, Middle East respiratory syndrome coronavirus (MERS-CoV) , severe acute respiratory syndrome coronavirus (SARS-CoV) , adenovirus, hepatitis B virus, hepatitis C virus, etc. Arbidol can induce the production and release of endogenous interferons and activate macrophages to participate in immune regulation. This compound exhibits a significant inhibitory effect against coronavirus under in vitro conditions.

Clinical Uses

1. Arbidol is used to prevent and treat upper respiratory tract infections caused by influenza A and B viruses.

2. It is a patented drug used to treat MERS-related infections and SARS-related infections.

3. It is recommended as an anti-COVID-19 drug in *the Guidelines for the Diagnosis and Treatment of COVID-19* (Tentative 7th Edition) .

Dosage and Administration

Guidelines for the Diagnosis and Treatment of COVID-19 (Tentative 7th Edition) recommends arbidol dosage of 200 mg each time for adults and 3 times a day, and the course of treatment not to exceed 10 d.

Adverse Effects

Mainly manifested as nausea, diarrhea, dizziness and increased serum aminotransferase.

Drug Interactions

Plasma protein binding rate of arbidol can reach 90%. Combination use with other drugs with high protein binding rate can produce competitive binding to plasma proteins, resulting in a significant increase in the free form of arbidol in peripheral blood. Clinically, the dose of arbidol should be adjusted with time.

Interferons

Interferons (IFNs) are broad-spectrum antiviral drugs belonging to a class of glycoproteins produced by monocytes and lympho-cytes in the body after viral infection.

Pharmacologic Effects and Mechanism

IFNs have a wide range of antiviral effects. In addition to blocking the invasion, amplification, release and other stages of the viral infection, IFNs also exert a certain blocking effect on re-infection and persistent infection by virus. After viral infection, cells can produce two subtypes of IFNs: IFN-α and IFN-β. They both play a strong antiviral role by stimulating immune cells such as lymphocytes, natural killer cells and macrophages. IFN-γ, another subtype of IFNs, is only produced and released by T lymphocytes and natural killer cell; therefore, it has a weak antiviral effect and a significant regulatory effect on immunity. Depending on the spe-cies, different viruses have their unique characteristics in various stages of infection, including invasion, uncoating, intracellular ampli-fication, assembly and release of virus particles. Accordingly, the targets and underlying mechanisms of IFNs for different viruses are different, and the antiviral effects of IFNs are also diverse. IFNs can induce the expression of protein kinase, oligoadenylate syn-thase, ribonuclease and other molecules, and manifest their antiviral effects after entering the cells. In 2013, Swiss scientists discovered that certain types of IFNs inhibit coronavirus replication in human respiratory epithelial cells. Meanwhile, in vitro studies also revealed that IFN-α and IFN-β have strong antiviral effects against MERS-CoV and SARS-CoV. These results provide a biological basis for the clinical applications of IFNs in COVID-19.

Clinical Uses

1. Antiviral effect   IFNs are broad-spectrum antiviral drugs and are mainly used for a variety of acute viral infectious diseases (including influenza, viral myocarditis, mumps, epidemic encephallitis B, etc.) and chronic viral infections (such as chronic active hepatitis B, cytomegalovirus infection, etc.) .

2. Anti-tumor effect IFNs exert their anti-tumor effects by inhibiting proliferation of tumor cells and enhancing immune function of patients. Currently, IFNs are widely used in cancer therapy.

3. Anti-COVID-19 effect IFN-α is recommended as an anti-COVID-19 drug in *Guidelines for the Diagnosis and Treatment of COVID-19* (Tentative 7th Edition) .

Dosage and Administration

Guidelines for the Diagnosis and Treatment of COVID-19 (Tentative 7th Edition) recommends IFN-α as an anti-COVID-19 drug. The dose is 5 million U or equivalent for each adult. The drug can be dissolved in 2ml sterilized water and applied by aerosol inhalation twice a day.

Adverse Effects

(1) The most common adverse reaction of IFNs is influenza-like syndrome, with which patients often have transient fever, chills, loss of appetite, headache, muscle pain, weakness, nausea and vomiting.

(2) Few patients after medication will suffer bone marrow suppression, abnormal liver function, kidney damage and other transient damages, which will subside after drug withdrawal.

(3) Be cautious of its toxic and side effects on the central and peripheral nervous systems, such as weakness, sleepiness, apathy, depression, and severe anxiety. Patients with mental illness should be prohibited.

Chloroquine

Chloroquine (CQ) is a synthetic 4-aminoquinoline derivative, and chloroquine phosphate is the phosphate form of chloroquine with enhanced chemical and biochemical stability.

Pharmacokinetics

CQ is rapidly and almost completely absorbed after oral administration, and the blood concentration reached the peak after 1~2 h, with approximately 55% of the drug in the plasma bound to nondiffusible plasma constituents. CQ is widely distributed in the body and it can pass through the membrane of red blood cells and accumulate in these cells. In case of invasion of malaria parasites into the red blood cells, high concentrations of CQ in these cells provide an important safeguard against malaria. CQ is metabolized by the liver with a $t_{1/2}$ of 50 h. CQ is excreted through the kidneys and its excretion is increased by acidification of urine, which can detoxify CQ poisoning.

Pharmacologic Effects and Mechanism

CQ kills plasmodium schizozoites inside red blood cells by inhibiting DNA replication, transcription and translation. However, CQ has no inhibitory effect on sporozoites, dormozoties and gametophytes during the quiescent period, so CQ does not prevent the spread of malaria. The concentration of CQ in the liver is significantly higher than that in blood. CQ can significantly kill Amoeba trophozoites implanted in the liver. CQ phosphate demonstrate certain curative effect on new coronary pneumonia in multi-center clinical studies.

Clinical Uses

1. Antimalarial effect   CQ is a highly effective agent against malaria, and prophylactic administration after entry into the affected area can suppress the onset of clinical symptoms of malaria.

2. Prophylactic administration   CQ can prevent the onset of malaria symptom. Therefore, CQ should be taken once a week during the period form 1 week before entering the affected area to 4 weeks after leaving the affected area.

3. Anti-parenteral amoebiasis   prescribed to patients with amoeba liver abscess.

4. Antiviral effect   CQ has inhibitory effects on a variety of viruses.

5. Immunosuppression effect   High doses of CQ and hydroxychloroquine can suppress immune responses in vivo. Hydroxychloroquine sulfate is used to treat autoimmune diseases such as systemic lupus erythematosus.

6. Anti-COVID-19 effect   CQ phosphate is recommended as an anti-COVID-19 drug in *Guidelines for the Diagnosis and Treatment of COVID-19* (Tentative 7th Edition) .

Dosage and Administration

CQ phosphate is suitable only for the treatment of *COVID-19* in adults aged 18~65 years. Suggested use: 500mg each time, twice a day for consecutive 7d for people who weigh more than 50kg. Note that a dosage of 500mg each time, twice a day for people who weigh less than 50kg, is recommended only for first two days, and from days 3~7, the dosage needs to be adjusted to 500mg, once/day. In addition, the dosage of CQ phosphate should be adjusted according to the patient's body weight during medication.

Adverse Effects

1. CQ over-dose can produce nausea, vomiting, dizziness, allergy and other adverse reactions. In order to effectively avoid adverse reactions, CQ can be used after meals.

2. Patients who have received long-term CQ therapy may experience visual disturbances or retinal edema. Initial and periodic ophthalmologic examinations should be performed. Patients with retinal or visual field changes are strictly restricted from taking CQ medication.

3. Rapid intravenous administration of CQ may cause hypotension. A high-dose CQ can inhibit the sinoatrial node. In some cases, CQ can lead to Adams-Stokes syndrome and even death. Patients with heart disease are strictly restricted. National Health Commission of the People's Republic of China published "Notice on the adjustment of the usage and dosage of CQ phosphate in the treatment of new coronary pneumonia" as a supplementary release, which requires monitoring ECG before using CQ phosphate. Only those with normal ECG can receive CQ phosphate treatment. Concomitant use of quinolones, macrolides and other drugs that can increase the QT intervals is contraindicated.

4. **Hearing damages**   CQ overdose for pregnant women may cause congenital deafness and baryencephalia in newborns. Hence, women in pregnancy and patients with hypoacusis or hearing loss are strictly restricted from taking CQ.

5. Patients with glucose-6-phosphate dehydrogenase deficiency are prohibited from taking CQ, for it may cause hemolytic anemia.

Drug Interactions

1. The inhibitory effect on the neuromuscular junction may be exacerbated when CQ phosphate is used in combination with streptomycin.

2. When combined with digitalis, CQ phosphate may slow cardiac electrical conduction, causing arrhythmias.

3. When combined with heparin or penicillamine, CQ phosphate may increase bleeding rate.

4. When combined with quinolones, macrolides, and other drugs that can prolong QT interval, CQ phosphate may cause further prolongation of QT interval, even leading to malignant arrhythmias.

Contraindications

National Health Commission of the People's Republic of China published "Notice on the adjustment of the usage and dosage of CQ phosphate in the treatment of COVID-19." The notice specifies the following taboos for CQ medication.

1. Pregnant women.

2. Patients who are allergic to 4-aminoquinoline compounds.

3. Patients with arrhythmias (conduction block) or chronic heart disease.

4. Patients with chronic malfunction of liver and kidney, particularly those reaching the terminal stage.

5. Patients with retinal disease, hypoacusis or hearing loss.

6. Patients with mental illness.

7. Patients with skin diseases (including rash, dermatitis, and psoriasis).

8. Patients with glucose-6-phosphate dehydrogenase deficiency.

9. Because of the underlying disease, patients who are taking the following medications are forbidden: drugs like digitalis, phenylbutazone, heparin, penicillamine, amiodarone, bepridil, domperidone, droperidol, haloperidol, azithromycin, astemizole, erythromycin, clarithromycin, posaconazole, methadone, procainamide, hydrochlorothiazide, sparfloxacin, levofloxacin, moxifloxacin, cis-

apride, indapamide, chlorpromazine, streptomycin, penicillamine, ammonium chloride, ondansetron, apomorphine, octreotide
monoamine oxidase inhibitor, and triamcinolone.

Ribavirin

Ribavirin (Virazole) is a synthetic guanosine derivative and a
broad-spectrum antiviral drug.

Pharmacokinetics

Ribavirin can be absorbed into the body by oral, aerosol, and
aqueous humor administrations and other means as well. The oral
absorption rate is rapid, and its bioavailability is about 45%. Plasma
concentration reaches the peak value after 1.5h of oral administration. Ribavirin is metabolized by liver and excreted by kidney. The
half-time ($t_{1/2}$) is 0.5~2h.

Pharmacologic Effects and Mechanism

Ribavirin is a broad-spectrum antiviral drug and it can inhibit a variety of RNA and DNA viruses (such as respiratory syncytial virus, herpes virus, influenza virus, hepatitis A virus, hepatitis C virus, Hantavirus, adenovirus, etc.) . Ribavirin is rapidly
phosphorylated when it enters virus-infected cell. Its phosphory-
lation products can be used as a competitive inhibitor of virus
synthetase and can inhibit a variety of key enzymes involved in
virus replication, thereby inhibiting the replication of virus RNA
and protein synthesis and ultimately block the proliferation and
release of virus. Ribavirin does not affect the process of virus adsorption, injection and uncoating, and not induce the production
of interferon in vivo either; thus, it has only a weak preventive
effect against virus infection. In vitro experiments showed that

ribavirin produces inhibitory effect on COVID-19.

Clinical Uses

1. It is employed to treat acute hepatitis A and C.

2. It is used to treat respiratory syncytial virus pneumonia, bronchitis and influenza.

3. It is recommended as a new anti-COVID-19 drug in *Guidelines for the Diagnosis and Treatment of COVID-19* (Tentative 7th Edition) .

Dosage and Administration

Guidelines for the Diagnosis and Treatment of COVID-19 (Tentative 7th Edition) recommends combined application of ribavirin and interferon or lopinavir/ritonavir via intravenous injection at a dosage of 500mg each time, 2 to 3 times a day for adults, and the course of treatment is not to exceed 10d.

Adverse Effects

1. Ribavirin accumulates excessively in red blood cells and it can cause anemia, asthenia and other adverse reactions. The symptoms disappear automatically after cessation of the drug administration.

2. Animal experiments showed that ribavirin has carcinogenic, teratogenic and mutagenic effects, and it can pass through the placental barrier and enter the milk. It is therefore restricted for pregnant and lactating women.

3. Ribavirin can cause myocardial damage in patients with anemia. Patients with a history of heart disease should be cautious when taking this drug.

Drug Interactions

Ribavirin can inhibit the transformation of zidovudine to zidovudine phosphate, and the combination of the two drugs can produce mutual antagonistic effects. For treatment of hepatitis C, ribavirin together with interferon can produce synergistic effect. *Guidelines for the Diagnosis and Treatment of COVID-19* (Tentative 7th Edition) suggests that ribavirin is to be used in combination with interferon or lopinavir/ritonavir to produce synergistic effects and to reduce the dose of ribavirin and increase antiviral activity with minimal adverse reactions.

HIV Protease Inhibitors

HIV protease inhibitors include ritonavir, nelfinavir, saquinavir, indinavir, amprenavir and lopinavir.

Pharmacologic Effects and Mechanism

Protease is one of the key enzymes in the process of HIV replication, which catalyzes the cleavage of HIV protein precursors and promotes the formation of structural proteins and the maturation and release of HIV virus. Protease inhibitors inhibit the cleavage of precursor proteins and the activation of immature non-infectious virus particles to manifest their antiviral effects.

The replication of coronavirus is similar to that of HIV virus, requiring catalysis by viral proteases. In vitro studies have shown that lopinavir and ritonavir can significantly inhibit the replication of MERS-CoV and SARS-CoV, suggesting their potential to resist coronavirus.

Clinical Uses

1. HIV protease inhibitors must be given in combination with other antiviral medications to produce a synergistic effect in treatment of HIV infection.

2. HIV infected adults who are not clinically suitable for treat-

ment with nucleoside or non-nucleoside reverse transcriptase inhibitors can be treated with HIV protease inhibitors alone.

3. Ritonavir and lopinavir are recommended as therapeutic drugs for COVID-19 in *Guidelines for the Diagnosis and Treatment of COVID-19* (Tentative 7th Edition) .

Dosage and Administration

Guidelines for the Diagnosis and Treatment of COVID-19 (Tentative 7th Edition) recommends that adults use lopinavir or ritonavir at a dosage of 200mg or 50mg/capsule, 2 capsules each time, twice a day for maximum 10d.

Adverse Effects

1. **Nervous system reactions** dizziness, headache, dull reaction, insomnia, abnormal taste.

2. **Gastrointestinal reactions** loss of appetite, anorexia, nausea, vomiting, abdominal pain, diarrhea.

3. **Allergic reactions** drug fever, dry skin, itching, drug rash, and skin erythema.

4. **Abnormal liver and kidney function.**

5. **Hematological reactions** spontaneous hemorrhage and hemolytic anemia.

6. **Metabolic response** insulin resistance, hyperglycemia, hyperlipidemia.

Drug Interactions

Protease inhibitors are mainly metabolized by hepatic cytochrome P450 and can interact with many other drugs that inhibit cytochrome P450 enzymes, thereby reducing their efficacy. The bioavailability of certain protease inhibitors in vivo changes with pH value. When used in combination with antacids, H_2 receptor antagonists, and proton pump inhibitors, the concentration of protease inhibitors in plasma can be reduced.

Favipiravir

Favipiravir is an RNA-dependent RNA polymerase inhibitor.

Pharmacokinetics

Favipiravir is well absorbed orally and has high bioavailability. The plasma protein binding rate of favipiravir in peripheral blood is 53%, and it is widely distributed in the body. Favipiravir is metabolized in liver and excreted through kidney.

Pharmacologic Effects and Mechanism

Favipiravir can be rapidly metabolized into favipiravir nucleoside triphosphate (M6) in vivo. M6 inhibits viral RNA-dependent RNA polymerase by mimicking guanosine triphosphate and the replication, transcription, and proliferation of viral genome. M6 can also insert into the viral genome to exert antiviral effects by inducing nucleotide mutations in the viral genome. In vitro experiments have shown that favipiravir has a significant inhibitory effect on coronavirus.

Clinical Uses

Currently, favipiravir has been approved for the treatment of new or recurring influenza in Japan. The United States has carried out Phase Ⅲ clinical trial of favipiravir for the treatment of influenza. Favipiravir has a strong inhibitory effect on many RNA viruses, such as Ebola virus, yellow fever virus, enterovirus, etc. This drug has recently obtained the drug registration approval for the treatment of COVID-19 in China and it is ready to be put into production for clinical application.

Adverse Effects

Increases blood uric acid, causes diarrhea, decreases neutrophil, and elevates liver transaminase.

Drug Interactions

The combination of favipiravir and pyrazinamide may increase the blood level of uric acid, and the combination of favipiravir and repaglinide may increase the blood concentration of repaglinide.

Remdesivir

Remdesivir is a prodrug of nucleoside analog with antiviral activity, belonging to the RNA-dependent RNA polymerase inhibitor.

Pharmacologic Effects and Mechanism

Remdesivir competes with ATP through a three-step conversion to the activated form of the triphosphate metabolite NTP and terminates the viral RNA transcription and amplification process after entering the cell in the form of prodrug. Preclinical studies have shown that remdesivir can suppress the replication and reproduction of the Ebola virus by inhibiting the RdRP protein of virus. Animal experiments have shown that remdesivir has pharmacological activity against MERS-CoV and SARS-CoV.

Clinical Uses

MERS, SARS, Ebola virus infection, and COVID-19.

Adverse Effects

This product has not been approved for marketing, and its safety and effectiveness have yet to be confirmed.

Triazavirin

The main active component of triazavirin is a synthetic analogue of purine nucleoside (guanine) base and has a wide range of antiviral effects on RNA containing viruses.

Pharmacologic Effects and Mechanism

Triazavirin can inhibit the synthesis and replication of viral RNA. The phase II clinical trail showed that triazavirin can shorten the duration of the main clinical symptoms (poisoning, fever, respiratory symptoms) , decrease the incidence of influenza related complications, and reduce the administration of symptomatic drugs. Triazavirin can be used to treat many other viral diseases, including tick-borne encephalitis. In addition, other studies showed that triazavirin has potential anti-Ebola effect. Recently, the clinical trial hosted by Yang Baofeng showed that triazavirin has a protective effect on COVID-19 patients, which can improve the clinical remission rate, shorten the course of treatment, promote the absorption of lung inflammation, increase the negative conversion rate of nucleic acid, and reduce the conversion rate of severe diseases. Triazavirin can improve the inflammatory reaction and hypercoagulability of the COVID-19 patients, reduce the incidence of complications in the course of treatment, and reduce the combination rate of drugs such as glucocorticoid usage and oxygen inhalation.

Clinical Uses

Influenza, Tick-borne encephalitis, Ebola virus infection, and COVID-19.

Adverse Effects

1. Allergy.

2. Gastrointestinal response: Bloating, diarrhea, nausea, vomiting, etc.

References

[1] BLAISING J, POLYAK S J, PÉCHEUR E I. Arbidol as a broad-spectrum antiviral: an update [J] . Antiviral Res, 2014, 107: 84-94.

[2] MOMATTIN H, MOHAMMED K, ZUMLA A, et al. Therapeutic options for Middle East respiratory syndrome coronavirus (MERS-CoV) -possible lessons from a systematic review of SARS-CoV therapy [J] . Int J Infect Dis, 2013, 17 (10): e792-798.

[3] CAMERON C E, CASTRO C. The mechanism of action of ribavirin: lethal mutagenesis of RNA virus genomes mediated by the viral RNA-dependent RNA polymerase [J] . Curr Opin Infect Dis, 2001, 14 (6): 757-764.

[4] FURUTA Y, KOMENO T, NAKAMURA T. Favipiravir (T-705) , a broad spectrum inhibitor of viral RNA polymerase [J] . Proc Jpn Acad Ser B Phys Biol Sci, 2017, 93 (7): 449-463.

[5] YANG B F, CHEN J G. Pharmacology [M] . 9th ed. Beijing: People's Health Press, 2018.

Hormonal drugs

Glucocorticoids

Glucocorticoids are among the most significant regulatory hormones in regulating stress response; meanwhile, it is also the most widespread used effective drug of choice for anti-inflammation and immunosuppression in clinic. The common glucocorticoids include prednisone, methylprednisolone, hydrocortisone and dexamethasone.

Pharmacokinetics

Glucocorticoids can be absorbed by oral administration and injection, and they are quickly metabolized in the liver by conjugation with a sulfate or glucuronic acid and secreted into the urine. The metabolic cycle of glucocorticoids is prolonged in patients with hepatic and renal insufficiency.

Pharmacologic Effects and Mechanism

1. Metabolism   Glucocorticoids stimulate several processes that collectively serve to regulate metabolism. Glucocorticoids increase the concentration of blood glucose through stimulating gluconeogenesis. They stimulate negative nitrogen balance through mobilization of amino acids from tissues. In addition to the stimulation of fat breakdown in adipose tissue, glucocorticoids can also cause salt and water retention, calcium suppression and phosphorus absorption.

2. Anti-inflammatory effects   Application of glucocorticoids can reduce the exudation of lymphocyte caused by alteration of telangiectasia and permeability, restrain capillaries and fibroblast proliferation, prevent the formation of conglutination and scar, and reduce inflammation sequelae.

3. Immunosuppressive effects   Glucocorticoids regulate the metabolism of nucleic acids in lymphocytes to inhibit the production and release of inflammatory cytokines by transforming the metabolism of intracellular and extracellular substances.

4. Anti-shock effect   Glucocorticoids improve the shock caused by the disturbance of microcirculation, the myocardial blood supply insufficiency and myocardial contraction disorder caused by vasospasm, and body's tolerance to bacterial endotoxin without any effect on the exotoxin by inhibiting the production of inflammatory factors and stabilizing the lysosomal membrane.

Clinical Uses

1. Infection and inflammation   Glucocorticoid is the drug of choice for treating acute toxic infection with shock. *Guidelines for the Diagnosis and Treatment of COVID-19* (Tentative 7th Edition) recommends the use of glucocorticoids in patients with progressive deterioration of oxygenation index, fast-moving iconography and overactive state of inflammatory response within the initial stage (3~5d) of onset. The recommended dose should not exceed the equivalent of methylprednisolone [1~2mg/ (kg·d)] . The application of glucocorticoids to the treatment of critical patients is effective. However, their application can also bring potential risks to patients (such as secondary infection and osteoporosis) . For the treatment of COVID-19 with glucocorticoid, it is necessary to accurately evaluate the disease progression of the patients, closely monitor the patient's vital signs, and actively search for alternative drugs or therapies.

2. Immunosuppression   Glucocorticoids can be used as the first-line drug to inhibit autoimmune diseases (such as rheumatic myocarditis) , and an adjuvant treatment of allergic diseases including bronchial asthma and anaphylactic shock to prevent alloimmunization caused by organ transplantation.

3. Anti-shock   Glucocorticoids can be used in combination with antibiotics to treat infectious poisoning shock caused by bacteria. For patients with complicated basic diseases, the treatment plan should be determined by multi-disciplinary consultation based on the clinical characteristics of the disease, and glucocorticoids should be used with caution or alternative drugs (therapy) should be selected.

4. Alternative medicine   Used for acute/chronic adrenocortical insufficiency or insufficient adrenocortical hormone secretion.

Adverse Effects

1. Iatrogenic adrenal hyperfunction   Long-term application of glucocorticoids is highly likely to cause metabolic disorders. The symptoms are usually moon faces, buffalo hump, edema, hypokalemia and hypertension.

2. Infection   Application of glucocorticoids can suppress inflammation and reduce symptoms. However, it also reduces the body's defense and repair functions at the risk of infection spreading and delaying wound healing.

3. Osteoporosis   Long-term application of glucocorticoids is often accompanied by decreased osteoblast activity, bone matrix decomposition and bone salt deposition disorders, eventually leading to osteoporosis. Application of glucocorticoid must be stopped in the presence of osteoporosis. During application of glucocorticoids, serum calcium and phosphorus content, urine calcium-creatinine ratio in an early morning urine sample, and markers of bone turnover (such as osteocalcin, urinary pyridinoline and deoxypyridinoline) should be closely monitored. Bone mineral density should be examined with imaging technologies.

4. Diabetes mellitus   Long-term use of glucocorticoids can cause disorders of glucose metabolism in patients with impaired glucose tolerance and diabetes.

5. Myocardial damage   Long-term application of glucocorticoids is likely to cause metabolic disorders, hypertension and atherosclerosis.

6. Peptic ulcer   Glucocorticoids stimulate gastric acid secretion, reduce gastrointestinal mucosal protection, and induce ulcers. Long-term use can also cause gastrointestinal bleeding or perforation.

7. Gestation   Application of glucocorticoid in pregnant women can induce cleft palate or stillbirth through the placenta.

8. Epilepsy   Long-term use of glucocorticoids can induce central nervous system diseases such as epilepsy or mental disorders. Overdose in children can well induce convulsion.

Drug Interactions

1. Glucocorticoid combined with nonsteroidal anti-inflammatory drugs can reduce gastric mucus secretion, promote protein decomposition, inhibit protein synthesis, and induce or aggravate

peptic ulcer and other diseases.

2. The combination of glucocorticoids and antidepressants aggravates the central nervous system diseases induced by glucocorticoids.

3. When glucocorticoids are used in combination with cardiotonic glycosides, they can induce arrhythmias possibly by causing water and sodium retention and potassium excretion.

4. Glucocorticoids when combined with carbonic anhydrase inhibitor can cause electrolyte metabolism disorder leading to severe hypokalemia, and the water and sodium retention caused by glucocorticoid can weaken the diuretic effect of diuretics.

5. The combination of glucocorticoids and immunosuppressants enhances the serious infection.

6. Using protein anabolic hormone with glucocorticoid increases the incidence of edema and induces or aggravates acne.

7. The combination of glucocorticoids and antituberculous drugs can reduce exudation and pleural adhesion.

References

[1] RUSSELL C D, MILLAR J E, BAILLIE J K. Clinical evidence does not support corticosteroid treatment for 2019-nCoV lung injury [J] . Lancet, 2020, 395 (10223): 473-475.

[2] YANG B F, CHEN J G. Pharmacology [M] . 9th ed. Beijing: People's Health Press, 2018.

Section III

Expectorants

Ammonium Chloride

Ammonium chloride belongs to a kind of stimulating expectorant.

Pharmacologic Effects and Mechanism

Oral administration of ammonium chloride can stimulate gastric mucosa and cause mild nausea. It also stimulates vagus to reflexively increase the secretion of respiratory glands and the osmotic pressure of the respiratory tract, which allow the water to seep into the respiratory tract to induce dilute sputum manifested by coughing.

Clinical Uses

1. To treat dry cough or sticky sputum not easy to be coughed out.

2. To acidify urine or correct metabolic alkalosis.

Dosage and Administration

Tablets are recommended to be dissolved in water and taken after meals.

1. **Adult (take orally)**　0.3~0.6g/time, 3 times a day. Diuresis, 0.6~2g/time, 3 times a day.

2. Children: 30~60mg/ (kg·d) , or 1.5g/m^2; evenly divided into 4 times.

Adverse Effects

1. Nausea, thirst or vomiting may occur after oral administration.

2. Overdose can cause high chlorosis acidosis, low blood potassium and low blood sodium.

Drug Interactions

1. Ammonium chloride is prohibited to combine with aureomycin, neomycin, macrodantin, sulfadiazine or warfarin. Additionally, it is not suitable to be combined with potassium excretion diuretic.

2. It should be avoided to combine with drugs which promote the excretion of alkaline drugs such as pethidine.

Contraindications

1. Patients allergic to ammonium chloride.

2. Patients with severe liver and renal insufficiency or ulcer disease.

3. Patients with metabolic acidemia.

Acetylcysteine

Acetylcysteine is a classical phlegm-dissolving drug that was first introduced in the 1960s.

Pharmacologic Effects and Mechanism

After being absorbed, the thiol group of acetylcysteine contained in the acetylcysteine molecule can break the disulfide bond in the sputum glycoprotein polypeptide chain and the DNA fiber in purulent sputum, resulting in a strong phlegm dissolving effect, thereby effectively reducing the viscosity of sputum and promoting sputum discharge so as to achieve effective treatment.

Clinical Uses

The drug has strong mucus dissolving ability and it is generally used for respiratory diseases characterized by excessive viscous secretions, such as acute bronchitis, acute attack of chronic bronchitis, bronchiectasis, chronic obstructive pulmonary disease, etc.

Dosage and Administration

1. Sparge   Used in non-emergency situations. It must be prepared as an aerosol by dissolving into 10% sodium chloride and applied via spray inhalation at 1~3ml/time, 2~3 times a day.

2. Drip into the trachea   5% solution for emergency; Drip through or directly into the trachea, 1~2ml/time, 2~6 times a day.

3. Intratracheal instillation   Injecting 5% solution from the periosteum of thyroid cartilage ring into the airway lumen by injector for emergency; 0.5~2ml/time (0.5ml/time for infants, 1ml/time for children and 2ml/time for adults) .

Adverse Effects

1. Nausea, vomiting, upper abdominal discomfort, diarrhea, cough and other adverse reactions occur occasionally which are generally relieved after drug reduction or stop. Rare allergic reactions such as rashes and bronchospasm.

2. Dripping too fast can cause side effects like nausea, vomiting, rash, itching, bronchospasm, dizziness, headache, fever and allergic reaction. Flushing, angioedema, tachycardia, hypotension and hypertension, erythrocytosis, leukopenia, pharyngitis, nasal (fluid) overflow, tinnitus happen sometimes. Slowing down the rate of intravenous drip can reduce the adverse reactions. Antihistamines are commonly used to counter these side-effects. Patients with se-

vere allergic reactions are advised to discontinue medication. Direct dripping into the respiratory tract can produce a large volume of sputa. Use sputum aspirator to attract sputum if necessary.

Drug Interactions

1. This product has compatibility contraindications with chymotrypsin, iodide oil and trypsin.

2. Combination with isoproterenol can enhance the efficacy and reduce adverse reactions.

3. Combination with nitroglycerin can enhance vasodilation function and delay tolerance but increase adverse reactions such as headache and hypotension.

4. Combination with antibiotics like penicillin, tetracycline and cephalosporin can weaken the antibacterial activity. Therefore, this medicine is generally not used in combination with these drugs. If necessary, it can be used alternately at intervals of 4h.

5. Combination with strong acid drugs significantly can reduce the efficiency of this drug significantly.

Bromhexine

Bromhexine is a sticky phlegm-regulating agent that can reduce the adsorption capacity of phlegm.

Pharmacologic Effects and Mechanism

Bromhexine exerts a strong phlegm-dissolving effect. After absorption, the compound can directly act on the phlegm-producing cells in tracheal and bronchial mucosa to lyse polysaccharide cellulose in sputum and dilute the sputum. It can inhibit the synthesis of goblet cells and mucous gland glycoprotein to reduce sialic acid and viscosity of sputum and promote cilia movement to facilitate sputum excretion.

Clinical Uses

Bromhexine has a dissolving effect. It is suitable for patients who have difficulty to cough out sticky sputum and patients with chronic bronchitis, emphysema, asthma, bronchiectasis, and silicosis. Patients with purulent sputum need antibiotics to control the infection.

Dosage and Administration

1. **Take orally**　8~16mg/time, 2~3 times/d.

2. **Subcutaneous, intramuscular, intravenous infusion or intravenous drip**　4~8mg/time, 1~2 times/d.

3. **Spray inhalation**　0.2%; 2ml/time, 1~3 times/d.

Adverse Effects

1. Mild adverse effects may be manifested as occasional nausea and stomach discomfort. A few patients may have temporary elevation of serum transaminase but can relieve by themselves.

2. Serious adverse effects may appear like rash, enuresis, etc.

Drug Interactions

It can increase the penetrability and concentration of amoxicillin and erythromycin in mucus. Clinical combination can enhance anti-infection effect.

Precautions

1. Patients who are allergic to the medicine are strictly restricted.

2. When using bromhexine cautions must be taken by patients with gastric ulcer and for pregnant and lactating women.

3. Children must be used under the supervision of adult, and the medicine should be kept out of the reach of children.

4. Taking after meals is recommended.

Qingfei Huatan Pill

Main Ingredients

Radix Scutellariae (roasted with Huangjiu) , *Semen Armeniacae Amarum, Semen Trichosanthis, Bulbus Fritillariae Cirrhosae, Rhizoma Arisaematis Cum Bile* (fried in sand) , *Rhizoma Pinelliae Preparatum* (fried in sand) , *Pericarpium Citri Reticulatae, Poria, Fructus Aurantii* (stir-frying with bran) , *Herba Ephedrae* (roasted with honey) , *Radix Platycodonis, Fructus Perillae*, roasted *Semen Raphani, Flos Farfarae* (roasted with honey) and *Radix Glycyrrhizae*.

Pharmacologic Effects and Mechanism

Radix Platycodonis produces its pharmacological effects and therapeutic efficacy by ventilating lung, eliminating phlegm, relieving sore throat and expelling pus, and has effects on symptoms such as cough with excessive phlegm, chest tightness, sore throat, aphonia, and lung carbuncle and pus. The main component of *Radix Scutellariae* is baicalin that is effective in clearing away heat and toxic materials, clearing away heat and dampness, and relieving spasm and it is used to treat hyperthermia, upper respiratory tract infection, cough with lung heat, etc. *Rhizoma Arisaematis Cum Bile* can clear away heat and phlegm, extinguish wind and arrest convulsion. The main component of *Semen Armeniacae Amarum* is amygdalin that can relieve cough, asthma, inflammation, analgesia, and loosen bowels and release constipation, and thus can be applied to manage cough, asthma, chest phlegm, blood deficiency and fluid deficiency. *Herba Ephedrae* is mainly composed of ephedrine that induces sweat and relieves asthma and diuresis, and it therefore can be used for relieving exterior syndromes such as fever, headache and body pain caused by exogenous wind cold. *Pericarpium Citri Reticulatae* can regulate Qi, invigorate spleen, regulate the middle warmer and dispel phlegm. *Flos Farfarae* (roasted with honey) is especially effective for chronic cough due to lung deficiency. Evidently, various ingredients in Qingfei Huatan Pill with reasonable compatibility work together to strongly descend Qi, eliminate phlegm and relieve cough and asthma.

Indications

Qingfei Huatan Pill is used for cough due to lung heat, excessive phlegm and asthma, excessive phlegm and saliva, and poor lung Qi.

Adverse Effects

Not yet reported.

Drug Interactions

This product contains *Herba Ephedrae*, the main component of which is ephedrine, which can cause certain reactions when applied in combination with other medicines.

1. It can enhance sweating and relieve exterior syndrome in combination with *Ramulus Cinnamomi*.

2. Combination with medicines containing tannins can precipitate ephedrine and reduce the therapeutic efficacy.

3. Combination with iron agent medicines can produce complexation reaction and reduce the therapeutic effects of iron agent.

4. Combination with monoamine oxidase inhibitors such as pargyline will cause hypertension crisis.

5. Combination with antihypertensive medicines can reduce the curative effects of antihypertensive medicines.

6. Combination with sedative hypnotics reduces the curative

effects of the latter.

7. Combination with aspirin and other antipyretic and analgesic medicines can cause sweating collapse.

8. Combination with isoniazid can cause dysuria.

Precautions

1. Avoid spicy and greasy food when taking Qingfei Huatan Pill.

2. Patients with bronchiectasis, lung abscess, pulmonary heart disease and pulmonary tuberculosis must seek the guidance of doctors.

3. During the course of treatment, if the target syndrome is not improved after taking the medicine for 3d, or in case of developing high fever with body temperature, dyspnea, or worsened coughs, and experiencing increased sputum volume, go and see a doctor immediately.

4. Children, pregnant women, and patients with weak constitution and spleen and stomach deficiency should use the medicine with caution.

5. Qingfei Huatan Pill contains *Radix Scutellariae* and can well cause allergy. Those who have allergic history on this medicine are highly restricted from taking this medicine.

6. Athletes should use it with caution.

References

LU L N, DONG J H, ZUO Y H, et al. Simultaneous determination of four components in Qingfei Huatan Pills by RP-HPLC [J] . Ready-for-use traditional Chinese medicine, 2016, 38 (09): 1956-1959.

Qutanling Oral Liquid

Main Ingredients

Qutanling Oral Liquid mainly contains fresh Bamboo Sap and *Herba Houttuyniae*, and the auxiliary materials include sucrose and sodium benzoate.

Pharmacologic Effects and Mechanism

Qutanling Oral Liquid can eliminate phlegm by promoting gland secretion, diluting sputum and accelerating bronchial endothelial cilia movement. It has an antitussive effect and can reduce cough duration. It has obvious inhibitory effects on *Staphylococcus aureus*, *Staphylococcus albus* and pneumococcus. It can improve the immunity of the body by enhancing the phagocytic function of macrophages and lymphocyte reactivity. It also has anti-inflammatory effects. *Herba Houttuyniae* has inhibitory effects on influenza virus, herpes simplex virus-1 (HSV-1) , human immunodeficiency virus-1 (HIV-1) and severe acute respiratory syndrome coronavirus (SARS-CoV) . In addition, it can also produce analgesic, diuretic and antioxidant effects.

Indications

Qutanling Oral Liquid generates its pharmacological effects and therapeutic efficacy by clearing away heat and toxic materials, resolving phlegm and relieving cough. Thus, it is mostly used for phlegm-heat cough indication that is characterized by cough, excessive phlegm, yellow and thick phlegm, and poor expectoration. Clinically, it is used to treat acute and chronic bronchitis and pneumonia with the above symptoms.

115

Adverse Effects

Adverse effects are not common and are relatively mild if any, which are mainly manifested as shortness of breath, laryngeal edema, chest tightness, palpitations, rash, etc. Fresh Bamboo Sap and *Herba Houttuyniae* are slightly cold plants, and children may occasionally experience thin and slightly increased stool and other symptoms.

Drug Interactions

Bamboo Sap contained in Qutanling Oral Liquid is compatible with ginger juice and suitable for phlegm-heat syndrome because it can reduce the disadvantages of cold stomach and intestine induced by Bamboo Sap.

Precautions

1. Patients who are allergic to this medicine are strictly restrained from taking it, and people with allergic constitution should use it with caution.

2. Pregnant women and weak people should use it with caution.

3. It is not suitable for subjects with cough of cold phlegm nature and loose stool due to spleen deficiency.

4. For patients who have high fever $\geq 38℃$ during medication with Qutanling Oral Liquid. Subjects who have apparent symptoms such as shortness of breath, wheezing, worsening cough, and increased sputum volume should immediately stop using this medicine and go to hospital.

References

[1] HONG Y M, CHEN C X, JIN R M, et al. Experimental study on

pharmacological effects of Qutanling Oral Liquid [J] . Shanghai Journal of Traditional Chinese Medicine, 1996, 06: 43-46.

[2] LIANG M H. Studies on the chemical constituents and pharmacological effects of *Herba Houttuyniae* [J] . Chinese Medicine Guide, 2019, 02: 153-154.

[3] LI J, ZHENG X S. Toxic mechanism of *Herba Houttuyniae* based on network analysis [J] . Journal of Shenyang Pharmaceutical University, 2019, 36 (11): 1047-1055.

[4] XU S G, LI M B. A summary of 150 cases of phlegm cough caused by Lung Heat in children treated with Qutanling Oral Liquid [J] . Shanghai Journal of Traditional Chinese Medicine, 1994, 12: 28.

Huatan Juhong Oral Liquid

Main Ingredients

Exocarpium Citri Grandis, *Radix Stemonae* (roasted with honey) , *Poria*, *Rhizoma Pinelliae* (prepared) , *Rhizoma Cynanchi Stauntonii*, *Radix Glycyrrhizae*, *Semen Armeniacae Amarum*, and *Fructus Schisandrae Chinensis.*

Pharmacologic Effects and Mechanism

Exocarpium Citri Grandis, *Rhizoma Pinelliae*, *Poria* and *Radix Glycyrrhizae* regulate Qi, eliminate dampness and phlegm. *Radix Stemonae* moistens lung and relieves cough. *Semen Armeniacae Amarum* and *Rhizoma Cynanchi Stauntonii* can ventilate lung Qi, descend Qi, eliminate phlegm and relieve cough. *Fructus Schisandrae Chinensis* can improve Qi. *Exocarpium Citri Grandis* has antitussive, expectorant, anti-inflammatory and bacteriostatic effects. *Exocarpium Citri Grandis* acts by eliminating phlegm, regulating Qi, invigorating spleen and promoting digestion, and is suitable for phlegm stagnation in chest, cough and asthma, food

117

stagnation, and vomiting and hiccup. *Radix Stemonae* offers antibacterial, antitussive, insecticidal, antiviral and other effects. *Poria* is used for cough due to phlegm drinking, phlegm-dampness entering collaterals, and shoulder and back pain. *Rhizoma Pinelliae* has the effects of eliminating dampness, eliminating phlegm, reducing retrogression and stopping vomiting. *Rhizoma Cynanchi Stauntonii* has the effects of reducing Qi, eliminating phlegm and relieving cough, and is used for lung Qi obstruction, cough with excessive phlegm, and chest fullness and dyspnea. *Radix Glycyrrhizae* has the effects of clearing away heat and toxic materials, treating cough with excessive phlegm, invigorating spleen and Qi, etc. The main component of *Semen Armeniacae Amarum* is amygdalin which can relieve cough, asthma, produce anti-inflammation and analgesia actions, and loosen bowels and relax constipation, and is therefore effective for cough, asthma, chest full phlegm, blood deficiency and fluid deficiency.

Indications

Huatan Juhong Oral Liquid acts to regulate Qi, eliminate phlegm, moisten lung and relieve cough. It can be used for cough, asthma and excessive phlegm caused by phlegm obstruction of lung, common cold, bronchitis and pharyngolaryngitis characterized by the above syndromes.

Adverse Effects

Not yet reported.

Contraindications

Not recommended for wind-heat patients.

Drug Interactions

Drug interactions may occur when used simultaneously with other medicines. Consult a doctor or pharmacist for details before taking this medicine.

Precautions

1. Smoke, wine and spicy, raw, cold and greasy food should be avoided during the course of medication with this medicine.

2. It is inappropriate to take nourishing traditional Chinese medicine during the course of taking this medicine.

3. Subjects who develop high fever with body temperature $\geqslant$ 38.5 ℃ , asthma and shortness of breath occur, cough worsening and sputum volume increasing significantly during the medication period it must discontinue and go to hospital.

4. Patients who have bronchiectasis, lung abscess, pulmonary heart disease and pulmonary tuberculosis and are coughing are urged to go to see a physician.

5. Patients with diabetes or severe chronic diseases such as hypertension, heart disease, liver disease and kidney disease should get advice from doctors prior to taking the medicine.

6. Children, pregnant women, lactating women, the elderly and the infirm should take it under the guidance of doctors.

7. If the target symptoms do not relieve after taking the medicine for 3 d, go and see a physician.

8. People who are allergic to this medicine are restrained from further medication with it, and people with allergic constitution should use it with caution.

9. Avoid using the medicine if it has deteriorated.

10. Children must use it under the supervision of adults.

References

[1] DAI J, FENG L, SUN M, et al. Determination of Morphine in

Juhong Huatan Pills by HPLC [J] . Journal of Pharmaceutical Analysis, 2008, 28 (10): 1757-1759.

[2] SITU W L, CHEN L, LI H B, et al. Determination of Naringin in Juhong Huatan Pills by RP-HPLC [J] . Journal of Guangdong Pharmaceutical University, 2015, 31 (1): 43-45.

[3] WANG Y H, HUANG J W, JIANG X, et al. Pharmacodynamics study on antitussive, phlegm-resolving, antiasthmatic and anti-inflammatory effects of Juhongtan Cough Liquid [J] . World Science and Technology-Modernization of Traditional Chinese Medicine, 2017, 19 (8): 1375-1380.

Section IV

Traditional Chinese Medicine

Jinhua Qinggan Granules

Jinhua Qinggan Granules is a medicine formulated based on the classic prescriptions "Maxing Shigan Decoction" and "Yinqiao Powder" and developed in China for battling influenza virus after the outbreak of influenza A (H1N1) in 2009.

Main Ingredients

Flos Lonicerae, Gypsum Fibrosum, Herba Ephedrae (roasted with honey) , *Semen Armeniacae Amarum, Radix Scutellariae, Fructus Forsythiae, Bulbus Fritillariae Thunbergii, Rhizoma Anemarrhenae, Fructus Arctii, Herba Artemisiae Annuae, Herba Menthae*, and *Radix Glycyrrhizae.*

Pharmacologic Effects and Mechanism

The basic prescription "Maxing Shigan Decoction" contained in Jinhua Qinggan Granules was originally formulated by ancient Chinese doctor Zhang Zhongjing specifically for clearing lung heat. When entering the lung meridian, *Herba Ephedrae* acts by dispelling lung heat. When combined with temperate *Gypsum Fibrosum* with cold and cool nature, Yinqiao Powder, *Flos Lonicerae* and *Fructus Forsythiae* for clearing heat and toxic materials, *Herba Menthae* pungent for dispersing exterior pathogens, and *Fructus Arctii* and *Radix Glycyrrhizae* for blending various medicine, Jinhua Qinggan Granules can produce curative effects on cough and asthma caused by lung heat.

Indications

It can be used for fever, mild or no aversion to cold, pharyngeal red and pharyngalgia, nasal obstruction and runny nose, thirst, cough or cough with phlegm, red tongue, thin yellow coating, rapid pulse and other symptoms caused by exogenous dampness. Jinhua Qinggan Granules is proven to be safe and effective in the treatment of influenza wind-heat invasion of lung syndrome. *Guidelines for the Diagnosis and Treatment of COVID-19* (Tentative 7th Edition) recommends Jinhua Qinggan Granules for patients with fatigue and fever during the medical observation period.

Adverse Effects

Nausea, vomiting, diarrhea, stomach discomfort, heartburn, poor appetite and other gastrointestinal adverse reactions can be seen. Occasional liver function abnormality, palpitation or rash.

Drug Interactions

Possible stomach irritation and gastrointestinal adverse reactions when Jinhua Qinggan Granules is taken together with anti-inflammatory and analgesic agents. Possible enhancement of myocardial excitability, cardiac output and heart rhythm when combined with cardiotonic glycosides. Possible promotion of vasoconstriction and induction of hypertension when combined with epinephrine.

Precautions

1. Avoid spicy, raw, cold and greasy food and adopt a light diet while taking the medicine.

2. *Herba Ephedrae* in Jinhua Qinggan Granules contains ephedrine as the main component, which is an epinephrine-like agent and could possibly constrict blood vessels, relax the bronchial smooth muscle, stimulate central nervous system, and aggravate cardiovascular diseases. Patients with hypertension, cardiac insufficiency, glaucoma, and immune deficiency should use it with caution.

3. The medicine contains *Gypsum Fibrosum* which is cold and cool in nature. Caution must be taken for subjects with deficient and cold spleen and stomach. Besides, due to the hypertensive effects of ephedrine, pregnant women are restricted from using Jinhua Qinggan Granules.

4. Jinhua Qinggan Granules may accumulate and eventually produce toxic effects in patients with liver dysfunction. Therefore, patients with liver diseases or abnormal liver function should use it with caution.

5. The medicine contains *Flos Lonicerae* and *Fructus Forsythiae* which can possibly cause allergy. Thus, subjects with allergic history to the medicine should discontinue the medication, and subjects with allergic constitution should use the medicine with caution.

References

LI G Q, ZHAO J, TU Z T, et al. Treating Influenza Patients of Wind-Heat Affecting Fei Syndrome by Jinhua Qinggan Granule: a double-blinded randomized control trial [J] . Chinese Journal of Integrated Traditional and Western Medicine, 2013, 33 (12): 1631-1635.

Huoxiang Zhengqi Capsule (Pill, Liquid, Oral Liquid)

Huoxiang Zhengqi Capsule (pill, liquid, oral liquid) is a Chinese patent medicine commonly used in clinics for the treatment of a wind-cold common cold.

Main Ingredients

Herba Pogostemonis, Folium Perillae, Radix Angelicae Dahuricae, Rhizoma Atractylodis Macrocephalae (parched) , *Pericarpium Citri Reticulatae, Rhizoma Pinelliae Preparatum, Cortex Magnoliae Officinalis* (made of ginger) , *Poria, Radix Platycodonis, Radix Glycyrrhizae, Pericarpium Arecae, Fructus Jujubae,* and *Rhizoma Zingiberis Recens.*

Pharmacologic Effects and Mechanism

Herba Pogostemonis produces its pharmacological activities by dispelling filth, eliminating dampness, and regulating the middle warmer. *Folium Perillae* has the effects of dispelling cold, regulating Qi, nurturing nutrients, promoting Qi circulation, harmonizing the middle warmer, and stopping vomiting. *Rhizoma Atractylodis Macrocephalae* has the effects of invigorating Qi and spleen, eliminating dampness, promoting diuresis, and stopping perspiration. *Pericarpium Arecae* has the effects of promoting Qi circulation, guiding stagnation, and regulating Qi. *Radix Angelicae Dahuricae, Poria* and *Radix Glycyrrhizae* have the effects of invigorating spleen and regulating stomach.

Modern pharmacological studies have found that Huoxiang Zhengqi Recipe has the following pharmacological functions:

1. Spasmolysis   Huoxiang Zhengqi Capsules, Pills, Powders, or other dosage forms produces inhibitory effects on gastrointestinal spasm.

2. Analgesia   Huoxiang Zhengqi Liquid has analgesic effects on visceral and somatic reflex pain caused by mesenteric injury in animal experiments.

3. Improving gastrointestinal dysfunction, bidirectionally regulating gastrointestinal motility, promoting digestion and absorption, relieving gastric distension, diarrhea, and controlling vomiting, enhancing intestinal absorption, and promoting the repair of gastrointestinal injury.

4. Enhancing cellular immune function and producing antibacterial and antiviral effects on *Sarcina luteus*, *Staphylococcus aureus*, *Shigella dysentery*, *Salmonella*, *Proteus*, *Trichophyton rubrum*, *Trichophyton Gypsum Fibrosum*-like, *Epidermis flocculus*, *Microspore Gypsum Fibrosum*-like, *Candida albicans*, *Cryptococcus neoformans*, *Bacillus dermatitis* and *Paratyphoid bacilli* A and B.

5. Anti-type I allergic reaction by inhibiting the release of allergic medium to improve the allergenic reaction of patients with the susceptible constitution.

Indications

It can be used to treat exogenous wind-cold, internal injury, and dampness, headache, diaphragmatic fullness, abdominal distension and pain, vomiting and diarrhea. It is suitable for the treatment of digestive, respiratory, endocrine system, pediatrics, dermatology, neurology diseases, and other diseases. Huoxiang Zhengqi Capsule is recommended by *Guidelines for the Diagnosis and Treatment of COVID-19* (Tentative 7th Edition) for

125

patients with fatigue and gastrointestinal discomfort during the medical observation period.

Adverse Effects

1. Systemic adverse effects, such as facial flushing, disulfiram-like reactions, allergic reactions, hypoglycemia, etc.

2. Adverse effects in the nervous system, including convulsions, dysphoria, coma, and headache.

3. Adverse effects in the cardiovascular system, such as palpitation and accelerated heartbeat, etc.

4. Adverse skin effects, such as medicine eruption, pruritus, etc.

5. Other rare adverse effects, such as visual damage, digestive system and respiratory system damage.

Drug Interactions

1. Huoxiang Zhengqi Capsule combined with levofloxacin in the treatment of acute gastroenteritis can enhance antipyretic and anti-diarrheal effects, relieve abdominal pain and promote the relief of clinical symptoms of patients.

2. Jiawei Huoxiang Zhengqi Pill combined with norfloxacin can improve the clinical symptoms of acute gastroenteritis with enhanced therapeutic effects.

3. Combination of Huoxiang Zhengqi Oral Liquid and loratadine offers improved therapeutic efficacy and safety in patients with chronic urticaria.

4. Huoxiang Zhengqi Liquid contains alcohol and when used together with cephalosporins, sedative-hypnotics, or antipyretic analgesics can cause disulfiram-like reactions and should therefore be avoided.

5. Huoxiang Zhengqi Capsules (pills, liquid, oral liquid) con-

tain *Herba Pogostemonis*, *Folium Perillae* and other dampness-removing and cold-dispelling medicines. The following nourishing traditional Chinese medicine should be avoided during the medication period.

Qi-supplementing medicine: *Radix Ginseng, Radix Codonopsis, Radix Pseudostellariae, Radix Panacis Quinquefolii, Radix Astragali seu Hedysari, Rhizoma Dioscoreae, Radix Glycyrrhizae*, etc.

Blood-supplementing medicine: *Colla Corii Asini, Fructus Lycii, Radix Polygoni Multiflori, Radix Angelicae Sinensis, Radix Rehmanniae Preparata*, etc.

Yin-supplementing medicine: *Bulbus Lilii, Radix Ophiopogonis, Herba Dendrobii, Radix Asparagi, Radix Glehniae, Radix Adenophorae*, etc.

Yang-supplementing medicine: *Cordyceps, Cortex Eucommiae, Herba Epimedii, Cornu Cervi Pantotrichum, Radix Morindae Officinalis*, etc.

Nourishing Chinese patent medicine includes Renshen Jianpi Pill, Buzhong Yiqi Pill, Qiju Dihuang Pill, Liuwei Dihuang Pill, Wuji Baifeng Pill, Shiquan Dabu Pill, etc.

Precautions

1. Patients with severe chronic diseases such as hypertension, heart disease, liver disease, diabetes and kidney disease, patients receiving other treatments or pregnant women should take Huoxiang Zhengqi Capsule medication under the guidance of doctors.

2. Children, the elderly and the physically weak should take it under the guidance of doctors.

References

[1] LI T N. Analysis of 108 cases of adverse reactions caused by Huoxiang Zhengqi Liquid (Dropping pills, Capsule, Granules) [C] . Hospital Pharmacy Committee of Chinese Pharmaceutical Association. Proceedings of the 23rd National Conference of pediatric pharmacy. 2012: 313.

[2] LIU S S, XIE Y M. Literature analysis of 101 cases of adverse reactions induced by Huoxiang Zhengqi Liquid [J] . Chinese Journal of Pharmacovigilance, 2017, 14 (05): 317-320.

[3] WANG P Y. Clinical study of Huoxiang Zhengqi Capsule combined with Levofloxacin in the treatment of 39 patients with acute gastroenteritis [J] . Modern Medical Imagelogy, 2019, 28 (05): 1186-1187.

[4] LI Y. Clinical study on the efficacy of norfloxacin combined with Jiawei Huoxiang Zhengqi Pill in the treatment of acute gastroenteritis [J] . Capital Food Medicine, 2019, 26 (18): 67.

[5] LIAO J M. Effect of Huoxiang Zhengqi Oral Liquid combined with loratadine on chronic urticaria [J] . Guide of China Medicine, 2019, 17 (32): 174-175.

Lianhua Qingwen Capsule (Granule)

Lianhua Qingwen Capsule is a broad-spectrum antiviral drug developed in 2003 for combating SARS.

Main Ingredients

Fructus Forsythiae, Flos Lonicerae, fried *Herba Ephedrae,* fried *Semen Armeniacae Amarum, Gypsum Fibrosum, Radix Isatidis, Rhizoma Dryopteris Crassirhizomae, Herba Houttuyniae, Herba Pogostemonis, Radix et Rhizoma Rhei, Herba Rhodio-*

lae, Menthol, and *Radix Glycyrrhizae*.

Pharmacologic Effects and Mechanism

Fructus Forsythiae, one of the main components of Lianhua Qingwen Capsule (Granule) , tasting cool and bitter can produce detoxifying effects to eliminate carbuncle, and thus used for treating the fire of upper energizer. Supplemented by menthol, *Radix Glycyrrhizae* can dispel cold and dissipate heat. *Flos Lonicerae* has the effects of resisting pathogenic microorganisms and clearing away heat and toxic materials and eliminating inflammation. *Herba Houttuyniae* has the effects of clearing away heat and toxic materials, eliminating carbuncle and discharging pus. Lianhua Qingwen Capsule (Granule) is effective for the syndrome of heat-toxicity attacking the lung.

Lianhua Qingwen Capsule (Granule) can also moderately relieve cough, eliminate phlegm and regulate immunity. In vitro studies show that this medicine not only has an anti-SARS effect, but also has certain inhibitory effects on influenza virus, parainfluenza virus type 1, respiratory syncytial virus, adenovirus types 3 and 7, herpes simplex virus types 1 and 2, *Staphylococcus aureus*, hemolytic streptococcus A and B, pneumococcus, *Haemophilus influenzae*, etc. Lianhua Qingwen Capsule inhibits the aggregation of macrophages into the lung tissue of rats with acute radiation-induced lung injury by inhibiting the expression of chemokines and reducing inflammatory reaction.

Indications

Lianhua Qingwen Capsule can be used for treating influenza, a syndrome of heat-toxicity attacking the lung. The symptom is manifested by fever or high fever, aversion to cold, muscle soreness, nasal obstruction and runny nose, cough, headache, dry throat and sore throat, red tongue, yellow or greasy coating, etc. It can also be used to treat acute pharyngitis and acute tonsillitis. In addition, it offers curative effects on acute respiratory tract infection, chronic obstructive pulmonary disease, viral keratitis, influenza, pneumonia, hand-foot-mouth disease, herpes zoster, pharyngitis, and herpes simplex. *Guidelines for the Diagnosis and Treatment of COVID-19* (Tentative 7th Edition) recommends it for patients with fatigue and fever during the medical observation period.

Adverse Effects

Acute diarrhea is occasionally seen, which is mainly manifested as gastrointestinal reactions, stomachache, stomach discomfort, nausea, vomiting, abdominal distension, and diarrhea. There are possible adverse reactions of skin system such as rash and pruritus.

Drug Interactions

Combined application of Lianhua Qingwen Capsule and cefuroxime in the treatment of acquired pneumonia can improve the therapeutic effects and shorten the time for symptom elimination, hospitalization and leukocyte recovery of patients. The combination of Lianhua Qingwen Capsule and Jingqiaomai Tablet produces rapid and safe curative effects on influenza A (H1N1). The combined application of Lianhua Qingwen Capsule and meropenem yields a synergistic effect on carbapenem-resistant *Acinetobacter baumannii*.

Precautions

1. Patients who are taking Lianhua Qingwen Capsule medication should avoid smoking, alcohol and spicy, raw, cold and greasy food and adopt a light diet.

2. The medicine is not suitable for the wind-cold common cold. Nourishing traditional Chinese medicine, especially warming

and tonifying traditional Chinese medicine must be avoided during Lianhua Qingwen Capsule medication.

3. Lianhua Qingwen Capsule contains *Herba Ephedrae* of which the main component ephedrine can likely cause contraction of blood vessels and stimulation of the central nervous system. Patients suffering from hypertension and heart disease and athletes should use it with caution.

4. The medicine contains *Radix et Rhizoma Rhei* and *Gypsum Fibrosum* which possess strong cold nature and can purge fire and relax constipation. Children, pregnant women, lactating women, the elderly and infirm, and people with spleen deficiency and loose stool should take it under the guidance of doctors.

5. Liver and kidney dysfunction can disturb the excretion of the medicine causing accumulation leading to toxicity. Patients with serious chronic diseases such as liver disease, diabetes, and kidney disease should take it under the guidance of doctors.

6. The medicine contains *Flos Lonicerae*, *Fructus Forsythiae,* and *Herba Houttuyniae* which can likely cause allergy. Subjects with allergic history to the medicine, or with allergic constitution should use it with caution.

References

[1] LEI Z, LU H D, DONG K C, et al. Lianhua Qingwen Capsules Inhibited the expression and effect of MCP-1 in rats with radiation-induced acute lung injury [J] . Herald of Medicine, 2014, 33 (07): 845-849.

[2] ZHANG Y F, TANG S W, WANG H R, et al. Effect of Lianhua Qingwen Capsules on inflammatory factors in mice with acute lung injury [J] . Food and Drug, 2015, 17 (02): 96-99.

[3] FENG Y. Clinical effect of Lianhua Qingwen Capsule combined

with Cefuroxime in the treatment of community acquired pneumonia [J] . Renowned Doctor, 2020, (01): 236.

[4] GUO W M. Clinical observation of Lianhua Qingwen Capsule joint with Jingqiaomai Tablet in treatment of influenza A (H1N1) [J] . Journal of Chengdu Medical College, 2015, 10 (03): 357-359.

[5] SHI L K, WANG Y, DONG X, et al. In vitro antibacterial experiment of Lianhua Qingwen Capsules combined with Meropenem against drug-resistant strains [J] . Chinese Journal of Nosocomiology, 2019, 29 (08): 1172-1175.

Shufeng Jiedu Capsule (Granule)

Shufeng Jiedu Capsule (Granule) is originated from Hunan folk secret prescription "Qudu Powder" and evolved from the original six ingredients to the present eight-ingredients formula. By rational compatibility with various traditional Chinese medicines, it acquires the ability to relieve exterior syndrome and clears away heat and toxic materials, and it has been used to treat seasonal plague, tonsillitis, mumps, pharyngitis, bronchitis, and chronic obstructive pulmonary diseases.

Main Ingredients

Rhizoma Polygoni Cuspidati, *Fructus Forsythiae*, *Radix Isatidis*, *Radix Bupleuri*, *Herba Patriniae*, *Herba Verbenae*, *Rhizoma Phragmitis*, and *Radix Glycyrrhizae*.

Pharmacologic Effects and Mechanism

Rhein, emodin and resveratrol in *Rhizoma Polygoni Cuspidati*, rosin in *Fructus Forsythiae* and saikosaponin in *Radix Bupleuri* produce their pharmacological activities by clearing away heat and toxic materials, promoting gallbladder and diuresis, removing yellow, and dispelling wind. *Herba Patriniae* and *Radix Isatidis* also have the effects of clearing away heat and toxic materials. *Radix Glycyrrhizae* plays a role in clearing away heat and regulating the body.

Shufeng Jiedu Capsule has certain inhibitory effects on influenza A virus H1N1, respiratory syncytial virus, herpes simplex virus, Coxsackie virus, etc. In addition, Shufeng Jiedu Capsule can reduce the level of inflammatory factors, thereby reducing the generation of heat-causing medium and exerting antipyretic effects. Forsythin, verbenin, emodin, verbascoside and some other components contained in the medicine have anti-inflammatory effects. The mechanisms of actions include reducing the level of inflammatory factors in serum and increasing the proportion of $CD4^+/CD8^+$ and NK lymphocytes, and activating the immune regulation process. It has therapeutic effects on pneumonia caused by acute pharyngitis and *Streptococcus pneumoniae*.

Indications

It is mainly used for treating acute upper respiratory tract infection, a wind-heat syndrome with symptoms including fever, aversion to wind, sore throat, headache, nasal obstruction, turbid nasal discharge, cough, etc. It can also be applied to respiratory diseases such as influenza and upper sensation. In addition, Shufeng Jiedu Capsule improves airway remodeling and nasal symptoms of allergic rhinitis-asthma syndrome (wind-heat invading lung syndrome) in patients with chronic obstructive pulmonary disease. Moreover, Shufeng Jiedu Capsule also has therapeutic effects on psoriasis vulgaris, hand-foot-mouth disease, herpes zoster, and other diseases. *Guidelines for the Diagnosis and Treatment of COVID-19* (Tentative 7th Edition) recommends it for patients with fatigue and fever during the medical observation period.

Adverse Effects

Occasional gastrointestinal symptoms, such as nausea, vomiting, abdominal pain, abdominal distension, etc. Occasional allergic rash, dizziness, headache, elevated blood pressure, facial redness and swelling, iris congestion, etc.

Drug Interactions

1. Combination with recombinant human interferon α-1b for the treatment of herpetic angina in children can reduce the fever duration, accelerate herpes regression, relieve pain and improve the therapeutic effects.

2. Combination with budesonide atomization improves clinical symptoms and inflammatory reactions in patients with acute pharyngitis.

3. Combination with levofloxacin hydrochloride tablets for the treatment of an acute attack of chronic bronchitis can rapidly relieve clinical symptoms and reduce inflammatory factors to improve clinical efficacy.

Precautions

1. Patients who are receiving Shufeng Jiedu Capsule (Granule) medication should avoid smoking, alcohol and spicy, raw, cold and greasy food and adopt a light diet life.

2. The medicine contains *Flos Lonicerae*, *Fructus Forsythiae*, *Radix Isatidis,* and other ingredients, which are clinically verified to be susceptible to cause allergy. It is forbidden for those with the allergic history of the medicine ingredients, and patients with allergic constitution should use it with caution for those.

3. When using this medicine, if you need to take other medicines, please consult the pharmacist first.

References

[1] LIU J, MA L, LU J, et al. Study on mechanism for antipyretic effects of Shufeng Jiedu Capsule [J] . Chinese Traditional and Herbal Drugs, 2016, 47 (12): 2040-2043.

[2] YANG Y, LI D Y. Therapeutic effect of Shufeng Jiedu Capsule combined with Recombinant Interferon α-1b on herpetic angina [J] . Journal of Emergency in Traditional Chinese Medicine, 2019, 28 (05): 899-900.

[3] ZHU S M, MAO X P, LIU Q. Clinical observation on the treatment of acute pharyngitis (Wind Heat Syndrome) with Shufeng Jiedu Capsule combined with budesonide atomization [J] . Medical Innovation of China, 2019, 16 (08): 67-71.

[4] YIN Z P, SUN S. Clinical study on Shufeng Jiedu Capsules combined with Levofloxacin in treatment of acute exacerbation of chronic bronchitis [J] . Drugs & Clinic, 2018, 33 (11): 2880-2883.

Fangfeng Tongsheng Pills (Granules)

Fangfeng Tongsheng Pill (Granule) is the upgraded form of the former "Fangfeng Tongsheng Powder" which was originated from *Clear Synopsis on Recipes* in *Yellow Emperor's Internal Classic-Plain Questions*. It has antipyretic, anti-inflammatory, and antibacterial effects through boosting up the immunity via dual actions: dispelling wind-cold outside and clearing heat inside.

Main Ingredients

Radix Saposhnikoviae, Herba Schizonepetae, Herba Menthae, Herba Ephedrae, Radix et Rhizoma Rhei, Natrii Sulfas, Fructus Gardeniae, Talcum, Radix Platycodonis, Gypsum

Fibrosum, *Rhizoma Ligustici Chuanxiong*, *Radix Angelicae Sinensis*, *Radix Paeoniae Alba*, *Radix Scutellariae*, *Fructus Forsythiae*, *Radix Glycyrrhizae* and *Rhizoma Atractylodis Macrocephalae* (parched) .

Pharmacologic Effects and Mechanism

Fangfeng Tongsheng Pill relieves exterior syndrome, dredges interior, and clears away heat and toxic materials. *Radix Saposhnikoviae* contained in this medicine possesses antipyretic, anti-inflammatory, antibacterial and immune-enhancing effects. *Herba Ephedrae* offers antipyretic, anti-inflammatory and analgesic effects. *Herba Schizonepetae* mainly contributes to counteracting bacteria, suppressing inflammation, lowering fever, promoting hemostasis, reducing cold, and elimination carbuncle. *Radix Platycodonis* relieves skin injury caused by allergic inflammation. *Radix Paeoniae Alba* elicits anti-inflammatory actions. At the molecular level, Fangfeng Tongsheng Pill increases the levels of $CD4^+/CD8^+$ in patients with chronic idiopathic urticaria and improves cellular immune function.

Indications

Fangfeng Tongsheng Pill is used to treat external cold and internal heat, exterior and internal excess, aversion to cold and improve heat function, headache and dry throat, short and red urine, constipation, rubella, and wet sores. It has certain curative effects on obesity, urticaria, acne, eczema, dermatitis, pruritus, headache, conjunctivitis, psoriasis, furuncle, asthma and other diseases.

Adverse Effects

Occasional skin allergic reactions including rash, or frequent and unformed stool, which can be relieved after medicine withdrawal or reduction.

Drug Interactions

Fangfeng Tongsheng Pill combined with loratadine, deslorata-dine or mizolastine alleviates chronic urticaria and prevents its recurrence rate. Combined application with glycyrrhizin and vitamin E to treat nonalcoholic fatty liver can improve liver function and blood lipid index.

Precautions

1. During the period of Fangfeng Tongsheng Pills (Granules) medication, patients should avoid smoking, wine and spicy, raw, cold and greasy foods, fish, shrimp and other seafood, and adopt a light diet.

2. During the period of Fangfeng Tongsheng Pills (Granules) medication, patients should stop taking nourishing traditional Chinese medicine of supplementing Qi, blood, Yang, and Yin.

3. Liver and kidney insufficiency can decrease the excretion of the medicine to render its accumulation within body and cause toxic actions.

4. Patients with chronic diseases such as liver diseases, diabetes, and kidney diseases should take the medicine under the guidance of doctors.

5. Children, pregnant women, lactating women, the elderly and infirm, and patients with loose stool due to spleen deficiency should take the medicine under the guidance of doctors.

6. Patients with hypertension and heart disease history and athletes should use the medicine with caution.

7. Patients with the allergic constitution should use it with caution.

References

[1] ZHAO M, PENG Y Q, SHI J H, et al. Study on the treatment of chronic urticaria with Fangfeng Tongsheng Powder [J]. Chinese Journal of Ethnomedicine and Ethnopharmacy, 2017, 26 (04): 45-48.

[2] QU E R. Clinical effect of Fangfeng Tongsheng Pill combined with Loratadine in the treatment of chronic urticaria [J]. Continuing medical education, 2019, 33 (05): 156-157.

[3] MIN Y. Clinical study of Fangfeng Tongsheng Pill combined with Desloratadine in the treatment of chronic urticaria [J]. Modern Journal of Intergated Traditional Chinsed and Western Medicine, 2015, 24 (35): 3945-3947.

[4] WEN S W, YANG Z M, LV Y, et al. Therapeutic effect of Fangfeng Tongsheng Pill combined with Mizolastine on chronic urticaria [J]. Chinese Journal of Clinical Rational Drug Use, 2012, 5 (07): 77-78.

[5] HE Y F. Clinical study of Fangfeng Tongsheng Pill combined with Compound Glycyrrhizin in the treatment of non-alcoholic fatty liver disease [J]. Zhejiang Journal of Integrated Traditional Chinese and Western Medicine, 2019, 29 (03): 197-200.

Shuanghuanglian Oral Liquid (Powder Injection)

Shuanghuanglian Oral Liquid is a pure traditional Chinese medicine preparation composed of *Flos Lonicerae*, *Radix Scutellariae* and *Fructus Forsythiae*. This medicine acts by clearing away heat and toxic materials and clearing both the exterior and the interior. It therefore can reduce swelling and relieve pain, resist infections by a broad spectrum of viruses and bacteria and improve the immune function of body.

Main Ingredients

Flos Lonicerae, *Radix Scutellariae* and *Fructus Forsythiae*.

Pharmacologic Effects and Mechanism

1. Antibacterial effects Shuanghuanglian Oral Liquid produces pronounced inhibitory effects on *Staphylococcus aureus*, *Proteus*, *Escherichia coli*, *Pseudomonas aeruginosa* and *Streptococcus pneumoniae*. The mechanisms mainly include direct disruption of the cell structure of bacteria, reduction of endotoxin, enhancement of immune function, interference with the formation process of bacterial biofilm, and inhibition of microbial enzyme activity and the activity of bacterial efflux pump.

2. Antiviral effects Shuanghuanglian Oral Liquid is a broad-spectrum antiviral medicine, and it has impressive anti-SARS coronavirus, anti-influenza virus (H7N9, H1N1, H5N1) , anti-SARS-CoV, anti-MERS-CoV and anti-Coxsackie virus effects. After the outbreak of COVID-19, cellular experiments conducted in Shanghai Institute of Medicine and Wuhan Institute of Virus demonstrated that Shuanghuanglian Oral Liquid has significant inhibitory effects on coronavirus. *Radix Scutellariae* in Shuanghuanglian can purge fire and detoxify, clear lung heat, and enhance the activity of natural killer cells (NK) , contributing to the antiviral efficacy of the medicine. *Flos Lonicerae* can clear away heat and toxic materials, cool blood, relieve sore throat, improve phagocytosis of leukocytes and inhibit virus proliferation. *Fructus Forsythiae* has antiviral effects by clearing away heat and toxic materials, reducing swelling and resolving hard mass, stimulating the production of interferon and immunoglobulin to fulfil its antiviral action.

3. Anti-inflammatory effects Shuanghuanglian Oral Liquid has strong antipyretic and anti-inflammatory effects. By inhibiting

vascular permeability, inflammatory cell synthesis and inflammatory factor secretion, it elicits anti-inflammatory effects.

4. Immune-boosting effect Shuanghuanglian Oral Liquid is a multifunctional immune enhancer, which can enhance human cell and humoral immune functions, and is therefore used for the treatment of infection.

Indications

1. Shuanghuanglian Oral Liquid is used for common cold caused by exogenous wind-heat with symptoms of fever, cough and sore throat.

2. Shuanghuanglian Oral Liquid has therapeutic effects on mild H1N1 epidemic upper respiratory tract infection, stomatitis and infantile mumps.

3. Shuanghuanglian Powder Injection is used for wind-warm disease with syndrome of pathogen invading lung-defense phase or syndrome of wind-heat invading lung. The symptoms include fever, slight aversion to wind-cold, cough and shortness of breath, yellow expectoration, red swelling and pain of pharynx. It is applicable to acute upper respiratory tract infection, acute bronchitis, tonsillitis and mild pneumonia caused by viruses and bacteria.

4. Shuanghuanglian Powder Injection has favorable clinical effects on acute urinary tract infection, severe mumps in children, viral encephalitis and hand-foot-mouth disease.

Adverse Effects

Common adverse reactions with Shuanghuanglian medication include rash, pruritus, angioneurotic edema, digestive system and nervous system diseases. Adverse reactions of digestive system are transient and can be removed after medicine withdrawal or routine treatment. Adverse reactions of respiratory and blood systems, high fever, chills, and anaphylactic shock often occur after intravenous administration.

Drug Interactions

Shuanghuanglian Oral Liquid combined with interferon atomization inhalation has significant effects on herpetic angina in children and can shorten the course of disease. Combination with ribavirin offers improved curative effects on mild epidemic upper respiratory tract infection of type A (H1N1) . When combined with penicillin, it is effective for respiratory tract infection in children. Taken along with ranitidine, Shuanghuanglian Oral Liquid can rapidly relieve the pain of ulcer patients, promote ulcer healing, and improve immune function.

Shuanghuanglian Powder Injection combined with conventional atomization inhalation can improve respiratory tract symptoms in patients undergoing tracheal intubation under general anesthesia. Combined with aciclovir, it can reduce the expression level of inflammatory factors in patients with viral encephalitis and achieve antiviral effects. Combined with ceftazidime, it can be used for the treatment of bronchopneumonia in children. Combined with cefepime, it may increase intracellular cefepime accumulation, causing cell damage and nephrotoxicity.

Shuanghuanglian Powder Injection often produces turbidity or precipitation when combined with aminoglycosides (gentamicin, kanamycin, streptomycin) , macrolides (erythromycin, leucomycin) , quinolones, etc.

Shuanghuanglian Oral Liquid contains traditional Chinese medicine with pungent and cool effects, and acts by relieving exterior syndrome, clearing away heat and toxic materials. Patients should not take the following nourishing traditional Chinese medicine while taking the medicine.

Qi-supplementing medicine: *Radix Ginseng, Radix Codonopsis, Radix Pseudostellariae, Radix Panacis Quinquefolii, Rhizoma Dioscoreae, Radix Glycyrrhizae*, etc.

Blood-supplementing medicine: *Colla Corii Asini, Fructus Lycii, Radix Polygoni Multiflori, Radix Angelicae Sinensis, Radix Rehmanniae Preparata*, etc.

Yin-supplementing medicine: *Bulbus Lilii, Radix Ophiopogonis, Herba Dendrobii, Radix Asparagi, Radix Glehniae, Radix Adenophorae*, etc.

Yang-supplementing medicine: *Cordyceps, Cortex Eucommiae, Herba Epimedii, Cornu Cervi Pantotrichum, Radix Morindae Officinalis*, etc.

Nourishing Chinese patent medicine include: Renshen Jianpi Pill, Buzhong Yiqi Pill, Qiju Dihuang Pill, Liuwei Dihuang Pill, Wuji Baifeng Pill, Shiquan Dabu Pill, etc.

Precautions

Evidence-based medical evidence for the treatment of COVID-19 with Shuanghuanglian (Oral Liquid, Powder Injection) is still lacking.

The precautions for Shuanghuanglian Oral Liquid include:

1. Avoid smoking, alcohol and spicy, raw, and cold and greasy food while taking the medicine.

2. Not suitable for people with cold.

3. Patients with diabetes, hypertension, heart disease, liver disease, kidney disease and other serious chronic diseases should take the medicine under the guidance of doctors.

4. Children, pregnant women, lactating women, the elderly and infirm, and patients with loose stool due to spleen deficiency

should use it under the guidance of doctors.

5. It is restricted for people who are allergic to this medicine, and caution must be taken for people with allergic constitution.

The precautions for Shuanghuanglian Powder Injection are as follows:

1. It is restricted for people who are allergic to this medicine, and caution must be taken for people with allergic constitution.

2. Patients with cough and asthma, severe angioneurotic edema, phlebitis, the elderly, the infirm, and patients with severe cardiopulmonary diseases should not take this medicine.

3. Do not take excessive dose or concentration (it is recommended that the concentration of liquid medicine should not exceed 1.2% during intravenous drip), especially for children, and the dosage should be calculated strictly according to body weight.

4. Intravenous drip of this product should follow the principle of slow beginning and fast follow-up: dripping should begin at 20 drops/min for 15~20 minutes and thereafter, if no discomfort is experienced, the dripping rate should speed up to 40~60 drops/min. Patient should be monitored for the possible appearance of adverse reactions.

5. Stop administering this product in case of turbidity or precipitation along with normal saline or 5%~10% glucose solution (the optimal pH value for this product is 6~8).

6. The first medication should be closely monitored. In appearance of rash, pruritus and facial congestion, especially palpitations, chest tightness, dyspnea, cough and other symptoms, the medication should be stopped immediately, and desensitization treatment needs to be initiated in time.

References

[1] GUO J, SONG D Y. Research progress in pharmacological action, clinical application and adverse reactions of Shuanghuanglian [J] . Chinese Journal of Clinical Rational Drug Use, 2017, 10 (21): 161-163.

[2] JIA J. Evaluation on the clinical application of Shuanghuanglian Oral Liquid [J] . Evaluation and Analysis of Drug-Use in Hospitals of China, 2013, 13 (02): 110-112.

[3] HUANG L. Effect of Shuanghuanglian Oral liquid combined with penicillin on upper respiratory tract infection [J] . Journal of Practical Traditional Chinese Medicine, 2018, 34 (05): 563-564.

[4] QIU J C, DIAO S G. Analysis of the curative effect of Shuanghuanglian Powder Injection combined with ceftazidime in the treatment of bronchopneumonia in children [J] . Jilin Medical Journal, 2014, 35 (12): 2548.

[5] LI A T, GU N B, TIAN Y, et al. Effect of Shuanghuanglian Injection on the expression of factors in viral encephalitis [J] . Shaanxi Journal of Traditional Chinese Medicine, 2015, 36 (09): 1109-1110.

Gelanxiang Oral Liquid

Gelanxiang Oral Liquid was launched in 2019. Its prescription is selected from the time-honored clinical prescription "Wugen Decoction". Gelanxiang Oral Liquid has the effects of clearing away heat, relieving exterior syndrome, and dredging internal heat. Modern pharmacological experiments revealed that Gelanxiang Oral Liquid has significant inhibitory effects on the proliferation of influenza virus related to respiratory tract infection in mice.

Main Ingredients

Radix Puerariae, Radix Isatidis, Rhizoma Phragmitis, Rhizoma Menispermi, Rhizoma Imperatae, Herba Pogostemonis, Flos Car-

thami, and *Radix et Rhizoma Rhei*.

Pharmacologic Effects and Mechanism

1. Anti-inflammatory effects and capillary permeability inhibition.

2. Antiviral effects   It inhibits the proliferation of influenza virus in lung.

3. Bacteriostasis   It has inhibitory effects on *Haemophilus influenzae* and *Klebsiella pneumoniae* in vivo. In vitro, it inhibits hemolytic streptococcus B, *Staphylococcus aureus*, *Candida albicans* and *Diplococcus pneumoniae*.

4. Antipyretic effects   It can inhibit the temperature rise caused by beer yeast in rats or by triple vaccine in rabbits.

Indications

It acts to clear heat, relieve exterior syndrome and dredge internal heat, and can be used for common cold, which is characterized by exogenous wind-heat and internal stagnation. The symptoms include fever, aversion to cold, head pain, nasal obstruction and runny nose, pharyngeal red and sore throat, dry mouth and thirst, abdominal distension and constipation, yellow urine, red tongue, thin white or yellow coating, and floating or slippery pulse.

Adverse Effects

Occasional stomach discomfort and diarrhea.

Drug Interactions

The following nourishing traditional Chinese medicines should be avoided while receiving Gelanxiang Oral Liquid medication.

Qi-supplementing medicine: *Radix Ginseng, Radix Codonopsis, Radix Pseudostellariae, Radix Panacis Quinquefolii, Radix Astragali seu Hedysari, Rhizoma Dioscoreae, Radix Glycyrrhizae*, etc.

Blood-supplementing medicine: *Colla Corii Asini, Fructus*

Lycii, Radix Polygoni Multiflori, Radix Angelicae Sinensis, Radix Rehmanniae Preparata, etc.

Yin-supplementing medicine: *Bulbus Lilii, Radix Ophiopogonis, Herba Dendrobii, Radix Asparagi, Radix Glehniae, Radix Adenophorae*, etc.

Yang-supplementing medicine: *Cordyceps, Cortex Eucommiae, Herba Epimedii, Cornu Cervi Pantotrichum, Radix Morindae Officinalis*, etc.

Nourishing Chinese patent medicine include: Renshen Jianpi Pill, Buzhong Yiqi Pill, Qiju Dihuang Pill, Liuwei Dihuang Pill, Wuji Baifeng Pill, Shiquan Dabu Pill, etc.

Precautions

1. Evidence-based medical evidence for the treatment of Gelanxiang Oral Liquid on COVID-19 is still lacking.

2. Patients should avoid smoking, alcohol and spicy, raw, cold and greasy food while taking the medicine.

3. It is not suitable for people with wind-cold.

4. Patients with diabetes, hypertension, heart disease, liver disease, kidney disease and other serious chronic diseases should take this medicine under the guidance of doctors.

5. Children, pregnant women, lactating women, the elderly and infirm, and patients with loose stool due to spleen deficiency should take this medicine under the guidance of doctors.

6. The medication period with this medicine should not last long: if the target symptoms do not disappear after 3 d, stop the medication and go to hospital.

7. People with physical weakness should use it with caution.

8. If sediment appears in Gelanxiang Oral Liquid, shake it before taking.

References

[1] LI Y, DONG L J, LI H X. Application of Wugen Decoction in pediatric heat syndrome [J] . Inner Mongolia Journal of Traditional Chinese Medicine, 2014, 33 (04): 67-68.

[2] ZHENG X P. A traditional Chinese medicine composition, preparation method and application. ZL200710130194.7 [P] . 2011-7-27.

Jinzhen Oral Liquid

Main Ingredients

Capra Hircus Cornu, Fritillaria Ussurensis Bulbus, Rhei Radix et Rhizoma, Radix Scutellariae, Chloriti Lapis, Gypsum Fibrosum, Bovis Calculus Artificial, and *Glycyrrhizae Radix et Rhizoma.*

Pharmacologic Effects and Mechanism

Capra Hircus Cornu can clear away heat, achieve sedative effects, dispel blood stasis and relieve pain, and can be used to relieve symptoms such as hyperthermia and excessive heat toxin. The main components of *Fritillaria Ussurensis Bulbus* are alkaloids, alkaloid glycosides, polysaccharides, volatile oils which have the effects of clearing heat, moistening lung, eliminating phlegm, relieving cough, relieving asthma, lowering blood pressure, etc. The effective components of *Rhei Radix et Rhizoma* are anthraquinones and anthrones which can attack accumulation and guide stagnation, promote blood circulation and remove blood stasis, purge fire and cool blood, clear away heat and dampness, and detoxify and eliminate carbuncle. *Radix Scutellariae* has antipyretic and detumescence effects, as well as broad-spectrum antiviral and antibacterial effects, and is effective for hyperthermia, upper respiratory tract infection, lung heat cough, etc. *Chloriti Lapis* can be applied to al-

147

leviate stubborn phlegm cementation, cough, dyspnea, chest tightness, and convulsion through its actions of dropping phlegm, lowering Qi, calming liver and relieving convulsion. *Gypsum Fibrosum* is pungent, cool and it can ventilate lung Qi, clear heat, relieve asthma and promote fluid. *Glycyrrhizae Radix et Rhizoma* is used to harmonize stomach and spleen, moisten lung, and detoxify and harmonize various medicines. Rational compatibility with various traditional Chinese medicines can clear away heat and toxic materials, eliminate phlegm and relieve cough.

Indications

It is used for children with acute bronchitis that conforms to phlegm-heat cough, manifested by fever, cough, cough and vomiting yellow phlegm, non-smooth cough and vomiting, red tongue, and yellow and greasy coating.

Adverse Effects

Occasional loose stool after taking the medicine, which disappears after stopping the medication.

Drug Interactions

1. This product should not be combined with Chinese patent medicine containing *Aconitum carmichaelii* Debx and *Aconitum kusnezoffii* Reichb.

2. *Rhei Radix et Rhizoma*, an ingredient of Jinzhen Oral Liquid, should not be combined with the following medicines: nuclear xanthic acid, nicotinic acid, caffeine, theophylline, ferralia, digitalis, pepsin, multi-enzyme tablets, tetracycline, rifampicin, sulfonamides, vitamin B_1, vitamin B_2, nicotinic acid, vitamin B_6, vitamin C; phenobarbital, sulfanilamide, penicillin, compound aspirin, medicinal charcoal, tannic acid protein, and alkaline medicines. Phentolamine can antagonize the hemostatic effects of the former; Chlo-

ramphenicol can reduce the purgative effects of the form *Rhei Radix et Rhizoma*, and isoniazid can easily form tannate precipitation to reduce absorption.

3. *Radix Scutellariae*, another ingredient of Jinzhen Oral Liquid, should not be combined with digitalis cardiac glycoside, propranolol and penicillin.

4. *Bovis Calculus Artificial* contained in Jinzhen Oral Liquid should not be combined with sedatives, anesthetics, anticonvulsants, chloral hydrate, morphine, phenobarbital, epinephrine and atropine.

5. *Gypsum Fibrosum*, which is contained in Jinzhen Oral Liquid, should not be combined with tetracycline, levodopa, erythromycin, rifampicin, prednisone, isoniazid, chlorpromazine and other medicines.

6. *Glycyrrhizae Radix et Rhizoma*, still another ingredient of Jinzhen Oral Liquid, should not be combined with Chinese patent medicines of *Kansui Radix*, *Euphorbiae Pekinensis Radix*, *Genkwa Flos* or *Sargassum* and hypoglycemic western medicine.

Precautions

1. Avoid spicy, raw, cold and greasy food during medication with Jinzhen Oral Liquid.

2. No nourishing traditional Chinese medicines should be taken during medication with Jinzhen Oral Liquid.

3. Patients with weak spleen and stomach and loose stool should use Jinzhen Oral Liquid with caution.

4. Patients with wind-cold closing the lung and long-term cough due to internal injuries should not use Jinzhen Oral Liquid.

5. Infants and diabetic children should take the medicine under the guidance of doctors.

6. During the medication period, if the patient does not experience any improvement of the relevant symptoms after 3d, or if the patient has high fever with body temperature exceeding 38.5℃ , go to hospital in no delay.

7. Subjects with allergic history to the ingredients of this medicine or with allergic constitution must take this medicine with caution.

References

LI J. Progress in clinical research and application of Jin Zhen Oral liquid [J] . Inner Mongolia Traditional Chinese Medicine, 2014, 33 (08): 118-119.

Xiyanping Injection

Main Ingredients

Andrographolide sulfonated compounds.

Pharmacologic Effects and Mechanism

Xiyanping Injection has inhibitory effects on influenza virus and respiratory syncytial virus. It also inhibits gram-positive bacteria such as *Dysentery bacilli*, *Pneumococcus*, and *Typhoid bacilli*. In addition, it has antipyretic effects on fever caused by bacterial or viral infection. This medicine can relax smooth muscle, relieve tracheal and bronchospasm, and produce antitussive effects. Moreover, it can also enhance the functions of various immune cells such as neutrophils and macrophages, promote the production of immunoglobulin, and improve immunity.

Indications

Xiyanping Injection is mainly used for bronchitis, tonsillitis, and bacillary dysentery. Several studies reported that Xiyanping

Injection is effective for patients with mild influenza and it can also be combined with azithromycin to treat mycoplasma pneumoniae pneumonia. It has been included in *Guidelines for the Diagnosis and Treatment of COVID-19* (Tentative 7th Edition) and can be used for patients with severe COVID-19 alone or complicated with mild bacterial infection.

Adverse Effects

Adverse reactions are primarily manifested in skin and its accessory system, gastrointestinal system, cardiovascular system and nervous system.

1. Allergic reactions are the most common adverse effects of Xiyanping Injection medication, mainly manifested as skin flushing, rash, pruritus, dyspnea, suffocation, urticaria, maculopapule, and angioedema.

2. Systemic adverse effects such as chills, fever, hyperhidrosis, pain, fatigue and edema and adverse reactions in digestive system including nausea, vomiting, diarrhea, abdominal pain, abdominal distension, dry mouth, and stomachache.

3. Other adverse effects are uncommon, including chest pain, chest tightness, shortness of breath, cough and other respiratory discomforts. Adverse cardiovascular reactions include palpitation, tachycardia and arrhythmia. Dizziness, headache, vertigo, tinnitus and other adverse nervous system effects.

4. Adverse effects caused by Xiyanping Injection normally disappear after medicine withdrawal or symptom-targeted treatment.

Drug Interactions

Combination with cephalosporin antibiotics for injection or vitamin B_6 for injection can change the pH value of the injection. Combination with acyclovir for injection or with ganciclovir for injection will reduce the content of sulfonated compound E, the main active ingredient of Xiyanping Injection. Generally, Xiyanping Injection is not used together with other injections. If other intravenous medicines need to be used in combination, Xiyanping Injection should be used first, and the infusion tube must be flushed prior to dressing change.

Precautions

1. Patients with allergic history and allergic constitution should take caution with Xiyanping Injection, and patients allergic to *Herba Andrographis* preparation must not take Xiyanping Injection medication.

2. In order to avoid the possible serious consequences of adverse reactions, people over 75 should take extra caution with the medicine.

3. For the first use of Xiyanping Injection, the patients should be closely observed for the possible adverse reactions at the initial stage of medication. If abnormalities are found, stop the medication immediately and receive appropriate treatment of the problems.

References

[1] CUI J, SI F G. Research progress in clinical application of Xiyanping Injection [J] . Journal of Huaihai Medicine, 2018, 36 (03): 378-380.

[2] WANG Z F, ZHANG H C, XIE Y M, et al. Expert consensus on clinical application of Xiyanping Injection in the treatment of respiratory infectious diseases (adult version) [J] . China Journal of Chinese Materia Medica, 2019, 44 (24): 5282-5286.

[3] ZHAO Y L, DONG P X, ZHENG L Y, et al. Evidence-based safety assessment of Xiyanping Injection [J] . Drug Evaluation, 2017, 14 (11): 5-11, 61.

[4] CHEN Y Y, XIE Y H, LIAO X, et al. Systematic review of medication safety of Xiyanping Injection in conformity with indications of package inserts [J] . China Journal of Chinese Materia Medica, 2016, 41 (18): 3463-3472.

[5] ZENG J, WU H W, YANG Z J. Meta-analysis of the safety of Xiyanping Injection in clinical application [J] . Chinese Journal of Clinical Rational Drug Use, 2018, 11 (22): 84-86.

Tanreqing Injection

Main Ingredients

Radix Scutellariae, Bear Bile Powder, *Cornu Capra Aegagrus Hircus*, *Flos Lonicerae* and *Fructus Forsythiae*.

Pharmacologic Effects and Mechanism

Tanreqing Injection has anti-inflammatory, anti-virus, expectorant, antitussive, antipyretic, sedative, antiasthmatic and other effects. It has broad-spectrum anti-pathogenic microorganism effects, and can inhibit respiratory pathogenic bacteria such as *Streptococcus pneumoniae*, hemolytic streptococcus B, *Staphylococcus aureus*, *Haemophilus influenzae*, *Pseudomonas aeruginosa*, etc. It can eliminate phlegm, relieve cough, effectively relieve pulmonary interstitial edema, airway spasm, mental stress, dyspnea and other symptoms of asthma patients, and obviously relieve asthma, wheezing and other symptoms.

Indications

Tanreqing Injection is primarily used for respiratory diseases such as acute bronchitis, upper respiratory tract infection, acute pneumonia, lung abscess, emphysema, pulmonary fungal infection, chronic obstructive pulmonary disease, etc. It can also be used for hand-foot-mouth disease, measles, and sepsis. Tanreqing

153

Injection is also a recommended medicine for the treatment of the Middle East respiratory syndrome (MERS) , dengue fever and H7N9 avian influenza virus infection. It has now been included in *Guidelines for the Diagnosis and Treatment of COVID-19* (Tentative 7th Edition) as a medicine for severe and critical COVID-19 patients, especially for COVID-19 patients complicated with mild bacterial infection.

Adverse Effects

The most common adverse reactions are damages to skin and its accessory system, manifested as rash, skin pruritus, urticaria, maculopapule, etc. Adverse respiratory reactions are also common, such as dyspnea, shortness of breath and short breath. Occasional dizziness, nausea, vomiting, palpitation, fever, and chills might be seen.

Drug Interactions

1. Combination with cefoperazone injection to treat community acquired pneumonia and acute exacerbation of chronic obstructive pulmonary disease can shorten the course of disease without obvious adverse reactions.

2. Combination of the medicine and meropenem for injection to treat lung infection can reduce the adverse reactions of meropenem and the incidence of fungal infection.

3. Tanreqing Injection has poor compatibility stability with levofloxacin, gentamicin, amikacin and azithromycin injection in vitro and is not suitable for compatibility application.

4. The medicine should not be combined with injections containing acidic substances.

5. The medicine is incompatible with tetrandrine A injection and sequential infusion must not be conducted.

Precautions

1. People with allergic history to the medicine or allergic constitution should use it with caution.

2. Elderly patients with liver and kidney insufficiency and severe pulmonary heart disease with heart failure, pregnant women, infants under 24 months, and subjects with superficial cold syndrome are restricted from using Tanreqing Injection.

3. The incidence of adverse reactions in children taking Tanreqing Injection is rare, but children with allergic history should be more vigilant and should be closely observed during medication.

References

［1］ PAN P X. Pharmacology and clinical application of Tanreqing Injection [J] . Chinese Journal of Clinical Rational Drug Use, 2015, 8 (17): 174-175.

［2］ ZHAO N B, WANG D X, DU X H. New progress in clinical application of Tanreqing Injection in the treatment of respiratory diseases [J] . Journal of Emergency in Traditional Chinese Medicine, 2018, 27 (04): 740-742.

［3］ WANG L, HUANG C Y, ZHANG F, et al. Analysis of research status of Tanreqing Injection in 15 years [J] . Journal of Emergency in Traditional Chinese Medicine, 2020, 29 (01): 36-40.

［4］ WANG S Y, HUANG D H, WANG C G. Systematic analysis of 38 cases of adverse reactions to Tanreqing Injection [J] . Henan Traditional Chinese Medicine, 2019, 39 (02): 263-266.

［5］ ZHENG W, NIE H X, YING L Q, et al. Incompatibility between Tanreqing Injection and Tetrandrine Injection [J] . Today Nurse, 2016, (03): 79.

Xingnaojing Injection

Main Ingredients

Moschus, Radix Curcumae, Borneolum Syntheticum, and *Fructus Gardeniae.*

Pharmacologic Effects and Mechanism

Xingnaojing Injection is made from Angong Niuhuang Pill. It produces pharmacological activities by clearing heat for resuscitation, eliminating phlegm, detoxifying, and regulating central nervous system and circulation system.

1. Regulation of central nervous system　Muscone contained in *Moschus* can reduce vascular permeability, scavenge oxygen free radicals, resist normal pressure hypoxia, and reduce apoptosis of hippocampal nerve cells caused by cerebral ischemia reperfusion injury. *Moschus* can also excite respiratory center, increase arterial oxygen partial pressure, reduce carbon dioxide partial pressure and improve blood gas index. Xingnaojing inhibits the expression of inflammatory factors and vascular endothelin, reduces blood viscosity, improves microcirculation and protects brain ultrastructure. *Fructus Gardeniae* can cause dehydration and diuresis to relieve cerebral edema.

2. Cardiovascular protection　Xingnaojing Injection enhances the tolerance to myocardial hypoxia by affecting adrenoceptor activity. The *Radix Curcumae* contained therein can cooperate with *Moschus* and *Borneolum Syntheticum* to induce resuscitation, dredge the channels and collaterals, and reduce blood lipid and blood viscosity. *Fructus Gardeniae* contained in Xingnaojing Injection has antihypertensive effects and can improve metabolism of myocardial local vasoconstrictor substances, relieve balance of myocardial blood supply and oxygen supply, and repair damaged myocardial cells.

3. Antipyretic effect   Xingnaojing Injection has excellent antipyretic effects and lasting curative effects.

Indications

It can be used as an adjuvant treatment of hyperthermia coma, acute cerebral infarction, craniocerebral injury, tuberculous meningitis, alcoholism, subarachnoid hemorrhage and epilepsy. It is included in *Guidelines for the Diagnosis and Treatment of COVID-19* (Tentative 7th Edition) and is recommended for COVID-19 patients complicated with high fever and consciousness disorder and for patients with severe and critical COVID-19. The medicine should be used strictly according to the indications and should not be used continuously for longer than 14d.

Adverse Effects

The side effects of Xingnaojing Injection are mostly chest tightness, dyspnea, accelerated breathing and other respiratory adverse reactions. Occasionally, allergic reactions such as rash, urticaria and flushing, as well as chills, fever, headache, dizziness, nausea and vomiting may appear.

Drug Interactions

Traditional Chinese medicine injection has complex components and high sensitization. It is strictly prohibited to mix Xingnaojing Injection with other traditional Chinese medicine injections or western medicines. When Xingnaojing Injection is prepared with 5% glucose injection, its microparticles are significantly higher than 0.9% sodium chloride injection, and thus, 0.9% sodium chloride should be used as the dilution solution. Xingnaojing Injection has poor stability in solution with low pH value.

Precautions

1. People with allergic history to Xingnaojing Injection or with allergic constitution should use it with caution. For the first-time user of this medicine, injection must be slow and the possible reactions must be closely inspected.

2. Patients with liver and kidney dysfunction, children and the elderly should use it with caution. This medicine is strictly restricted for pregnant women.

3. Xingnaojing Injection strongly promotes blood circulation and removes blood stasis and thus combination with other similar medicines must be avoided.

References

［1］ XU Y H. Pharmacodynamic study and clinical application of Xingnaojing Injection [J] . Modern Journal of Integrated Traditional Chinese and Western Medicine, 2010, 19 (4): 507-509.

［2］ LIU Y, HUANG A Q, ZHOU H H, et al. Clinical effect of Xingnaojing Injection combined with Nimodipine in the treatment of subarachnoid hemorrhage [J] . China Modern Medicine, 2019, 26 (36): 93-95, 99.

［3］ CHEN X, WU S H, WEN J X, et al. Systematic evaluation of the clinical effect of Xingnaojing Injection in the treatment of tuberculous meningitis [J] . Evaluation and Analysis of Drug-Use in Hospitals of China, 2019, 19 (12): 1430-1434, 1440.

［4］ CAO H L. The application of hyperbaric oxygen combined with Xingnaojing Injection in the rehabilitation of patients with severe craniocerebral injury [J] . Modern Medicine&Health, 2020, 36 (02): 256-258.

［5］ CHEN Y, PEI G M. Comparative observation on insoluble particles of Xingnaojing Injection with different dilutions [J] . Hubei Journal of Traditional Chinese Medicine, 2016, 38 (3): 72-74.

Xuebijing Injection

Xuebijing Injection is a medicine for promoting blood circulation and removing blood stasis, which embodies the theory of warm disease treatment with traditional Chinese medicine for resisting heat-toxicity and static blood and poison. It is used to treat serious infectious diseases caused by inflammation, endotoxin and sequent organ failure.

Main Ingredients

Flos Carthami, Radix Paeoniae Rubra, Rhizoma Ligustici Chuanxiong, Radix Salviae Miltiorrhizae and *Radix Angelicae Sinensis*.

Pharmacologic Effects and Mechanism

Xuebijing Injection elicits its pharmacological effects and therapeutic efficacy by removing blood stasis and detoxifying. Modern pharmacology shows that Xuebijing Injection can reduce the level of endotoxin and antagonize the release of endogenous inflammatory mediators induced by endotoxin. It enhances the anti-oxidative stress capacity to minimize the oxidative stress-induced organ injuries. It can also correct immune response deficiency and boost immune function of the body. It can protect vascular endothelial cells, improve microcirculation, and help repair damaged organs under stress.

Indications

Xuebijing Injection can be used to treat the syndrome of static blood and poison in warm diseases, such as fever, asthma, palpitation and dysphoria. Clinical studies show that Xuebijing Injection has strong anti-endotoxin effects, reduces the level of pro-inflammatory factors and improves the level of anti-inflammatory factors. Xuebijing Injection is suitable for patients in the organ function damage phase of systemic inflammatory response syndrome and multiple organ dysfunction syndrome induced by infection. Xuebijing Injection can significantly improve immune function and inhibit non-specific immune hyperfunction, and thus can be used for improving immune dysfunction in sepsis. Xuebijing Injection can correct coagulation dysfunction, improve microcirculation, increase blood oxygen saturation and reduce organ failure under stress. *Guidelines for the Diagnosis and Treatment of COVID-19* (Tentative 7th Edition) recommends Xuebijing Injection as a therapeutic medicine against systemic inflammatory response syndrome and multiple organ failure in critical COVID-19 patients, which could possibly suppress inflammatory factors thereby inflammatory storm severe and critical COVID-19 patients. Combining it with antibacterial agents can effectively delay the pathological progression of severe COVID-19.

Adverse Effects

1. Respiratory symptoms   Patients may suffer from short breath, chest tightness, dyspnea and other symptoms, which are related to the purity and impurity residues of Xuebijing Injection.

2. Skin symptoms   Patients may have rash, pruritus and facial flushing.

3. Incidental digestive system symptoms and cardiovascular system symptoms are seen.

Drug Interactions

1. Direct compatibility with other injections is to be avoided during intravenous drip.

2. Some of the main active ingredients of Xuebijing Injection are the same as some other Chinese patent medicine preparations (such as Salvia Ligustrazine and Biqi Capsule) and they therefore should not be combined.

3. Xuebijing Injection should not be combined with antacid medicines, because tanshinone (the active ingredients in Xuebijing Injection) could form metal ion complexes with metal ions (Ca^{2+}, Al^{3+}, Mg^{2+}) in antacid medicines.

4. *Radix Salviae Miltiorrhizae* contained in Xuebijing Injection should not be combined with cytochrome C, vitamin K, strychnine, ephedrine, atropine and other medicines.

5. Xuebijing Injection combined with ulinastatin can effectively improve lung function and relieve symptoms of severe pneumonia.

6. Combination with antibiotics is used to treat severe lung infection, and such a combination significantly reduces inflammatory reaction without causing serious allergic reactions. No abnormalities are found in liver and kidney function, hematuria routine and other indicators.

7. Combination of Xuebijing Injection and dexamethasone can inhibit the inflammatory reaction and improve the clinical symptoms of sepsis.

Precautions

1. Xuebijing Injection contains *Flos Carthami* and invigorates the circulation of blood. It is forbidden for pregnant women and women in menstrual period. It should be used with caution for patients with abnormal coagulation function.

2. It should be used with caution for elderly patients and patients with liver and kidney dysfunction. Patients with other basic diseases should use it under the guidance of doctors.

3. Before medication, patients should be requested in detail about their allergic history and whether they have a history of adverse reactions to traditional Chinese medicine injections. Patients should strictly

follow the indications. Once adverse reactions occur, stop the medication immediately and seek medical treatment timely.

References

［1］ ZHANG S W, SUN C D, WEN Y. Effect of treatment with Xuebijing Injection on serum inflammatory mediators and Th1/2 of spleen in rats with sepsis [J] . Chinese Critical Care Medicine, 2006, 18 (11): 673-676.

［2］ Chen J, Zhang Y. Effect of Xuebijing Injection on patients with sepsis inflammatory reaction and coagulation function [J] . Journal of Hunan Normal University (Medical Sciences) , 2016, 13 (2): 105-107.

［3］ LI Z J, SUN Y Y, WU Y L, et al. Experimental study of protective effects of Xuebijing Injection on stress-induced organ damage in rabbit [J] . Chinese Critical Care Medicine, 2006, 18 (2): 105-108.

［4］ NIE A R, GUO Z K, ZHANG Y, et al. Literature analysis of 211 cases of adverse reactions of Xuebijing Injection [J] . Strait Pharmaceutical Journal, 2019, 31 (11): 246-249.

［5］ PANG J F, PAN X B. Clinical effect of Xuebijing combined with Ulinastatin in the treatment of severe pneumonia [J] . Chinese Community Doctors, 2019, 35 (9): 96-98.

［6］ YE Q. Clinical analysis of Xuebijing combined with Antibiotics in the treatment of severe pulmonary infection in ICU [J] . China Healthcare Innovation, 2013, 8 (14): 29.

［7］ LI C Y, ZHANG X Y, LIU S, et al. Novel coronavirus pneumonia (COVID-19) evidence and research prospect of Xuebijing Injection [J] . Modernization of Traditional Chinese Medicine and Materia Medica-World Science and Technology, 2020, 22 (2): 1-6.

Reduning Injection

Main Ingredients

Herba Artemisiae Annuae, Flos Lonicerae, and *Fructus Gardeniae*.

Pharmacologic Effects and Mechanism

Reduning Injection has significant pharmacological effects such as anti-inflammation, antivirus, antipyretic and analgesic, immune regulation, etc. Reduning Injection can significantly inhibit influenza virus, orphan virus, herpes virus, EV71 virus and various respiratory tract virus strains. In addition, Reduning Injection has obvious antibacterial effects: inhibiting various bacterial strains (such as *Staphylococcus aureus*, hemolytic streptococcus B, *Escherichia coli*, *Shigella*, *Vibrio cholerae*, *Typhoid bacillus*, *Paratyphoid bacillus*, etc.) and other pathogenic microbials (including *Streptococcus pneumoniae*, *Neisseria meningitidis*, *Pseudomonas aeruginosa* and *Mycobacterium tuberculosis*) . Reduning Injection has been shown to reduce the mortality rate of animals infected by *Staphylococcus aureus* and *Klebsiella pneumoniae* as well as the serum levels of inflammatory factors. Reduning Injection can also reduce fever and enhance immune function.

Indications

Reduning Injection can be used for cough, high fever, aversion to cold, headache and yellow phlegm caused by exogenous wind-heat, acute upper respiratory tract infection, acute bronchitis and pneumonia.

1. **Influenza**   Reduning Injection combined with oseltamivir and amantadine can reduce the body temperature of patients and accelerate fever reduction and symptom disappearance in patients with influenza A (H1N1) .

2. **Chronic bronchitis**   Reduning Injection combined with cefuroxime can treat chronic bronchitis.

3. **Pneumonia**   Reduning Injection combined with ribavirin can treat viral pneumonia and mycoplasma pneumonia in

children, accelerating disappearance of cough and pulmonary rales. When combined with levofloxacin for the treatment of community acquired pneumonia, this medicine relieves respiratory symptoms and promotes the recovery of leukocyte indexes. Combination with protective ventilation for the treatment of acute lung function injury significantly increases arterial oxygen partial pressure, delays disease progression and reduces mortality.

4. *Guidelines for the Diagnosis and Treatment of COVID-19* (Tentative 7th Edition) recommends Reduning Injection as an anti-COVID-19 therapeutic medicine for COVID-19 patients complicated with mild bacterial infection.

Adverse Effects

1. Volatile oils, organic acids, triterpene saponins and flavonoids contained in Reduning Injection are easy to form immune complexes in blood and cause allergic reactions. Patients may develop systemic redness, pruritus or rash, etc. In severe cases, anaphylactic shock may occur.

2. Reduning Injection can cause digestive system reactions, manifested as abdominal pain, diarrhea, stomachache, etc. Some patients, mainly children may develop dizziness, chest tightness, dry mouth, nausea, and vomiting.

Drug Interactions

1. Reduning Injection compatibility with cephalosporins such as cefazolin, cefuroxime, ceftriaxone and cefoperazone may lead to varying degrees of changes of user's appearance.

2. Reduning Injection will lose its stability after direct compatibility with quinolone antibiotics such as levofloxacin, gatifloxacin, moxifloxacin hydrochloride, etc.

3. Direct compatibility of Reduning Injection with aciclovir, ambroxol and metronidazole can generate microparticles. Reduning Injection should not be used together with other medicines. If combination is needed, the infusion tube should be flushed with 0.9% sodium chloride solution or administered at intervals prior to use.

4. The active components of Reduning Injection (geniposide, quercetin and chlorogenic acid) have certain effects on the activity of CYP enzyme. When combined with medicines metabolized by relevant CYP enzyme, the dosage should be re-adjusted.

Precautions

1. The medicine can cause allergic reactions and thus should be used with caution for people who are allergic to the medicine and those who have allergic history on traditional Chinese medicine injection. It should be used with caution for the elderly, children, pregnant women and patients with liver and kidney dysfunction.

2. The medicine can increase the levels of direct bilirubin and total bilirubin and therefore caution must be taken for patients with hemolysis history (slight increase of blood bilirubin or positive urinary bilirubin) .

3. Prior to taking Reduning Injection medication, patients must be requested to provide information on age and allergic history and the dosage and speed of infusion, and the course of treatment must be under strict control. Once adverse reactions occur, stop the medication immediately and seek symptomatic treatment thereafter.

4. Patients with other basic diseases should use it under the guidance of doctors.

References

[1] LUO X C. Pharmacological action, clinical application and adverse reactions of Reduning Injection [J]. Chinese Journal of Pharmacovigilance, 2013, 10 (4): 215-218.

[2] SHE J. A new antibacterial and antiviral drug-Reduning Injection [J]. Central South Pharmacy, 2010, 8 (7): 548-550.

[3] YANG H J, LI G S, WANG H Y. Adverse reactions of Reduning Injection [J]. Public Medical Forum Magazine, 2017, 21 (34): 4881-4882.

[4] MIAO Q. Adverse reactions and prevention of the Reduning Injection [J]. Clinical Journal of Chinese Medicine, 2017, 9 (22): 120-121.

[5] KANG D Y, GENG T, DING G, et al. Research progress of clinical combination and drug interaction of Reduning Injection [J]. China Pharmacy, 2017, 28 (2): 276-279.

Shengmai Injection

Shengmai Injection is developed according to the ancient prescription "Shengmai Powder". It is mainly used clinically for the rescue and treatment of critical diseases such as myocardial infarction, cardiogenic shock and septic shock.

Main Ingredients

Radix Ginseng Rubra, *Radix Ophiopogonis*, and *Fructus Schisandrae Chinensis*.

Pharmacologic Effects and Mechanism

Shengmai Injection produces its pharmacological effects and therapeutic efficacy by invigorating Qi, nourishing Yin, restoring pulse for relieving desertion, protecting cardiovascular function and regulating immunity.

1. Cardiovascular protection   Shengmai Injection has antioxidant stress and anti-inflammatory effects, enhancing myocardial tolerance to hypoxia and minimizing myocardial ischemia reperfusion injury. Shengmai Injection elevates the plasma level of tissue plasminogen, reduces blood and plasma viscosity, improves oxygen metabolism and hemodynamics. Shengmai Injection maintains normal blood pressure through its bidirectional regulatory mechanism (lowering hypertension and elevating hypotension) without affecting normal blood pressure of patients. Shengmai Injection can improve cardiac contractile function and cardiac output.

2. Lung protection   Shengmai Injection reduces arterial blood carbon dioxide partial pressure, increases arterial blood oxygen partial pressure and improves lung function.

3. Immune regulation   Shengmai Injection can reduce the serum levels of proinflammatory factors, relieve inflammatory reaction, and regulate immune function.

Indications

Shengmai Injection is used for the treatment of cardiovascular and cerebrovascular diseases and as an adjuvant treatment of acute pancreatitis, acute poisoning, tumors and other diseases.

1. Myocardial ischemia, myocardial infarction and heart failure   Shengmai Injection can reduce blood viscosity and improve angina pectoris and myocardial ischemia of coronary heart disease in elderly. Early application of Shengmai Injection after the onset of myocardial infarction can prevent the deterioration of myocardium and reduce the occurrence of complications. Shengmai Injection combined with nitroglycerin intravenous drip for the treatment of congestive heart failure can significantly increase left ventricular ejection fraction.

2. Pulmonary heart disease   Shengmai Injection combined with glucocorticoid intravenous drip can be used to treat pulmonary heart disease.

3. Tumor chemotherapy   Shengmai Injection reduces cardiac toxicity, hepatotoxicity, nephrotoxicity and acute toxicity caused by chemotherapy and improves chemotherapy compliance of patients.

4. Shengmai Injection is recommended as an anti-COVID-19 therapeutic medicine for critical COVID-19 patients in *Guidelines for the Diagnosis and Treatment of COVID-19* (Tentative 7th Edition) .

Adverse Effects

1. Allergic reactions, such as rash which may cause anaphylactic shock in severe cases.

2. Certain patients may suffer from digestive system damage after medication, such as abdominal distension and liver function damage.

3. Incidental cardiovascular system damage, such as palpitation, blood pressure drops, sinus tachycardia, sinus arrest, etc.

Drug Interactions

1. When the medicine is prepared with 0.9% sodium chloride and 10% glucose solution, it can alter pH and induce salting-out phenomenon of the solution, resulting in insoluble particles. Therefore, it is recommended to use 5% glucose solution as the solvent.

2. It is strictly prohibited to directly mix and match with other medicines. Combination with other medicines should be rationally guided with caution.

3. The medicine contains organic acid components and should

not be combined with aluminum hydroxide to avoid neutralization reaction and reduction of therapeutic action.

4. It is not suitable to be combined with nitrofurantoin, *p*-aminosalicylic acid, rifampicin, aspirin, phenobarbital, phenytoin sodium and indometacin, to avoid the possible toxic effects consequent to excessive concentration of the above-mentioned medicines in bloodstream.

5. The medicine can hinder the absorption of zinc and they should not be taken together.

6. The medicine contains tannins and to avoid the possible decreases in the pharmacological activities and therapeutic effects one should not be taken together with pancreatin and amylase.

7. The medicine contains *Radix Ginseng Rubra* which is not suitable for combination with *Veratri Nigri Radix et Rhizoma*, *Faeces Togopteri* and other medicines according to the incompatibility guide of traditional Chinese medicine.

Precautions

1. The medicine can produce adverse reactions such as allergy and is forbidden for newborns and infants. Patients with liver and kidney dysfunction, elderly patients, women in physiological period, pregnancy and childbirth, and patients with allergic constitution must take serious cautions on the medication.

2. Strictly follow the indications and monitor the medication. For the first-time application, the dosage of Shengmai Injection should not exceed 10~30ml to minimize the potential adverse reactions.

3. Patients with other basic diseases should use it under the guidance of doctors.

References

[1] YANG Z Q, AO J B, CAI L L, et al. Clinical study on Shengmai Injection in treatment of cardiogenic shock after acute myocardial infarction [J] . Drugs & Clinic, 2017, 32 (1): 20-24.

[2] XU S H, LIU S Y. Progress on pharmacological effect of Shengmai Injection [J] . Chinese Pharmaceutical Affairs, 2010, 24 (4): 405-407.

[3] LIAO M L, YU J, HUANG C B, et al. New progress in clinical application of Shengmai Injection [J] . West China Journal of Pharmaceutical Sciences, 2002, 17 (2): 152-154.

[4] WANG Y L, YUAN Y. Safety analysis of Shengmai Injection in clinical application [J] . Shanghai Medical & Pharmaceutical Journal, 2018, 39 (5): 38-43.

[5] TU C. Literature analysis of 38 cases of adverse reactions of Shengmai Injection [J] . Strait Pharmaceutical Journal, 2018, 30 (4): 266-268.

[6] FENG J, CAO J W, YAO J, et al. Study on the compatible stability of Shengmai Injection and common infusion [J] . Zhejiang Journal of Integrated Traditional Chinese and Western Medicine, 2016, 26 (1): 82-84.

Shenfu Injection

Shenfu Injection originates from "Shenfu Decoction" contained in *Ji Sheng Fang* (*Recipes for Saving Lives*) . It is a classic prescription of "restoring Yang, rescuing patient from collapse, and invigorating Qi for relieving desertion".

Main Ingredients

Radix Ginseng Rubra and *Radix Aconiti Lateralis Preparata* (black aconite tablet) .

Pharmacologic Effects and Mechanism

Shenfu Injection has cardiovascular and microcirculation

protective effects and immune regulatory effects as well, primarily through its ability to restore Yang, rescue patient from collapse and invigorate Qi for relieving desertion. Studies have shown that Shenfu Injection also has the following known or potential pharmacological functions:

1. **Anti-shock effects**　Shenfu Injection antagonizes hypotension caused by endotoxin and inhibits continuous decrease of peripheral arterial pressure. Shenfu Injection enhances right ventricular stroke volume, output per minute, ejection fraction and cardiac index and improves oxygen delivery and right ventricular function in patients with septic shock. Shenfu Injection improves blood viscosity, reduces platelet aggregation, increases peripheral blood perfusion, improves tissue metabolism, and increases blood supply and oxygen supply to brain tissue. Shenfu Injection protects vascular endothelial cells, relieves microcirculation vasospasm and improves microcirculation.

2. **Cardiac protection**　Shenfu Injection inhibits lipid peroxidation, reduces the level of reactive oxygen, improves the tolerance of myocardium to hypoxia, and improves impaired ultrastructure of myocardium. Shenfu Injection inhibits the expression of inflammatory factors and reduces inflammatory reaction. It can down-regulate the expression of proapoptotic protein, reduce myocardial cell apoptosis and reduce hypoxia-induced cardiac injury. It can increase myocardial contractility, slow down heart rate, reduce myocardial oxygen consumption, improve cardiac function and reduce ventricular arrhythmia.

3. **Protection of lung function**　Shenfu Injection can inhibit inflammatory reaction and reduce lung injury caused by endotoxin. Ginsenoside and water-soluble aconitine contained in Shenfu

Injection can relax bronchial smooth muscle, inhibit vasospasm, and reduce pulmonary vascular resistance and pulmonary artery pressure. Shenfu Injection reduces blood viscosity and erythrocyte aggregation, promotes fibrinolysis, reduces platelet aggregation, accelerates blood flow, improves microcirculation and alveolar ventilation, promotes the synthesis of pulmonary surfactant and improves oxygenation.

4. **Immune regulation**　Shenfu Injection promotes cellular immunity, stimulates spleen lymphocyte metabolism and enhances immune regulation and resistance to noxious stimulation. It can enhance the detoxification function of liver and directly resist liver and lung injury caused by endotoxin.

Indications

Shenfu Injection can be used for syndromes such as sudden Yang collapse, deficiency of both Qi and Yin, pulse deficiency and collapse, etc. , and is commonly used for shock, heart failure, coronary heart disease, and lung disease.

1. **Septic shock**　Combination of Shenfu Injection with conventional western medicines can improve microcirculation of patients with septic shock and significantly increase arterial blood pressure and central venous oxygen saturation of patients, reduce inflammatory reaction and improve hemodynamics in patients with septic shock. In *Guidelines for the Diagnosis and Treatment of COVID-19* (Tentative 7th Edition) , Shenfu Injection is recommended as an anti-COVID-19 therapeutic medicine for critical patients complicated with shock.

2. **Myocardial infarction complicated with heart failure**　Shenfu Injection combined with anticoagulants can reduce the level of inflammatory factors in patients with heart failure and im-

prove myocardial enzyme spectrum, cardiac function and prognosis of patients.

3. Chronic obstructive pulmonary disease　Conventional western medicine treatment combined with Shenfu Injection can increase the levels of immunoglobulin IgA, IgM and IgG in serum of patients with chronic obstructive pulmonary disease and enhance immune function.

Adverse Effects

1. Common adverse reactions are allergic reactions, such as flushing complexion, vexation and heat, dry mouth and tongue, etc.

2. Occasional serious adverse reactions may develop, such as chills, fever, cold limbs, salivation, blood pressure and heart rate drop, etc.

Drug Interactions

1. Shenfu Injection contains *Radix Ginseng Rubra* and *Radix Aconiti Lateralis Preparata*. According to the incompatibility guide of traditional Chinese medicine, it is not suitable to be used together with traditional Chinese medicine such as *Rhizoma Pinelliae, Fructus Trichosanthis, Bulbus Fritillaria, Radix Ampelopsis, Rhizoma Bletillae, Faeces Togopteri, Veratri Nigri Radix et Rhizoma*, etc.

2. Mixing Shenfu Injection with other medicines may produce insoluble particles, pH changes and flocculent precipitates. If combination is needed, the infusion pipeline should be flushed with 0.9% sodium chloride solution prior to infusion.

3. In the course of Shenfu Injection medication for patients with persistent angina pectoris, nitrate may be added under physician's advice.

4. The prescription contains black aconite tablet which should not be combined with hormones for a long period to avoid deficien-

cy of kidney Yin and loss of Yin essence in the body.

Precautions

1. The medicine can cause adverse reactions such as allergy and is therefore prohibited for patients with allergy or serious adverse reactions. The incidence of adverse reactions with Shenfu Injection medication is relatively low. Most of them occur in patients with allergic history, combined medication, over-indication, high dripping speed, high doses, prolonged duration of treatment, elderly and infirm patients and patients with basic cardiopulmonary diseases. Reactions of patients to the medicine need to be closely monitored, especially within the initial 30 minutes of infusion. Most of the adverse reactions caused by Shenfu Injection are common and mild, which will relieve or disappear upon withdrawal of the medication or with symptomatic treatment.

2. The composition of traditional Chinese medicine injection is complex and pregnant women, newborns and infants should not use it.

3. Patients with basic diseases should use it under the guidance of doctors.

References

［1］ XU J, LOU H G, LOU Y J, et al. Research progress in pharmacological action of "Shenfu Injection" [J] . Shanghai Journal of Traditional Chinese Medicine, 2008, 42 (10): 87-89.

［2］ Cao J H. Clinical analysis of Shenfu Injection in the treatment of septic shock [J] . China Foreign Medical Treatment, 2019, 38 (32): 121-123.

［3］ LIN H F. Clinical effects of Shenfu Injection combined with Xuebijing Injection on inflammatory index and hemodynamics in septic shock [J] . Journal of North Pharmacy, 2019, 16 (12): 51-52.

［4］ FENG J P, LIANG M F, WANG Y H, et al. Shenfu Injection combined with Enoxaparin Sodium in the treatment of acute myocardial infarction with heart failure [J] . Drug Evaluation Research, 2019, 42 (10): 2057-2061.

[5] WANG Z F, ZHAO W, ZHANG Y, et al. Analysis of influencing factors on adverse reactions of Shengfu Injection based on large prospective safety monitoring [J] . China Journal of Chinese Materia Medica, 2015, 40 (24): 4746-4749.

Shenmai Injection

Shenmai Injection is derived from Shendong Drink description in *Symptoms-Cause-Pulse-Treatment*. Its pharmacological effects and therapeutic efficacy are underlined by invigorating Qi for relieving desertion, nourishing Yin and promoting fluid production. It is a classic prescription of "strengthening vital Qi to eliminate pathogenic factors" in the theory of traditional Chinese medicine.

Main Ingredients

Radix Ginseng Rubra and *Radix Ophiopogonis*.

Pharmacologic Effects and Mechanism

Radix Ginseng Rubra invigorates spleen, lung, Qi and blood. *Radix Ophiopogonis* nourishes Yin, promotes fluid production, and moistens dryness. Shenmai Injection has the following known and potential pharmacological effects:

1. Cardiac protection Shenmai Injection protects the heart against oxidative stress injury, stabilizes mitochondrial membrane potential, reduces apoptosis with myocardial ischemia and hypoxia, reduces ischemic injury and improves cardiac function. It can stabilize cell membrane and maintain normal ion distribution inside and outside cells, enhance energy generation in ischemic region, improve coronary circulation and myocardial metabolism, and prevent ventricular arrhythmia. Shenmai Injection can activate β adrenoreceptors and inhibit Na^+-K^+-ATPase activity to enhance myocardial contractility. It inhibits renin-angiotensin-aldosterone system and improves heart failure.

2. **Anti-shock functions**   Shenmai Injection can increase blood pressure of hemorrhagic shock animals, excite adrenocortical system and promote reticuloendothelial system to remove various pathological substances. It can inhibit Na^+-K^+-ATPase activity of vascular smooth muscle cell membrane, promote Ca^{2+} influx, contract peripheral blood vessels, and increase blood perfusion of heart, liver, brain and other important organs. It can significantly improve the number of white blood cells, enhance the expression of IL-18 and interferon γ, resist infection of various pathogenic microorganisms, inhibit inflammatory reaction, and reduce systemic inflammatory response syndrome and multiple organ dysfunction syndrome caused by endotoxin.

3. **Immune regulation**   It can reduce lymphocyte apoptosis caused by endotoxin, promote the development of immune organs, enhance the phagocytosis of monocytes, increase the number of white blood cells, elevate the levels of plasma γ-globulin, IgG and IgM, and enhance the nonspecific immune function of the body.

4. **Improve pulmonary function**   Shenmai Injection increases diaphragm contractility, reduces diaphragm cell apoptosis, improves diaphragm diastolic function, reduces pulmonary artery pressure and pulmonary circulation resistance, and improves pulmonary ventilation and pulmonary gas exchange. It can reduce the levels of cytokines and neutrophil infiltration in lung tissue, block the binding of endotoxin to alveolar macrophage membrane, and reduce acute lung injury.

Indications

Shenmai Injection can be used for treating shock due to deficiency of both Qi and Yin and internal heat, coronary heart disease, viral myocarditis and chronic pulmonary heart disease.

1. **Shock**   Combined application of Shenmai Injection on the top of routine treatment of anaphylactic shock and traumatic shock can obviously improve the curative effects, shorten the duration of disease, rapidly blood pressure and control the pathological progression.

2. **Pulmonary heart disease**   Shenmai Injection can improve left ventricular systolic function of patients with pulmonary heart disease, improve blood viscosity and hypoxia symptoms of patients with chronic pulmonary heart disease, shorten the course of disease and reduce the occurrence of respiratory failure.

3. **Myocardial ischemia and heart failure**   Shenmai Injection can be used to prevent acute myocardial ischemia-reperfusion injury, reduce myocardial oxygen consumption, reduce infarct area, improve left ventricular ejection fraction, improve therapeutic efficacy, and reduce the development of complications such as hemorrhage and reperfusion arrhythmia. It can effectively treat congestive heart failure, improve clinical signs and cardiac function of patients with heart failure, and improve hemodynamics and microcirculation.

4. *Guidelines for the Diagnosis and Treatment of COVID-19* (Tentative 7th Edition) recommends Shenmai Injection as an anti-COVID-19 therapeutic medicine for critical COVID-19 patients.

Adverse Effects

Shenmai Injection can cause allergic reactions, such as dyspnea, asthma, cyanosis, cold limbs, salivation around the mouth, and anaphylactic shock in severe cases. Some patients can also suffer from skin damage and digestive system damage, such as rash, exfoliative dermatitis, abdominal pain, abdominal distension, etc. , and circulatory system symptoms, such as tachycardia and hypotension, etc. , which disappear or relieve after withdrawal of the medicine.

Drug Interactions

1. Shenmai Injection should not be used in combination with *Veratri Nigri Radix et Rhizoma, Faeces Togopteri* and their preparations.

2. Shenmai Injection should not be combined with glycerol fructose injection, penicillin and other high sensitivity medicines.

Precautions

1. The medicine can cause allergy and other adverse reactions and is strictly restricted for patients with allergy to *Radix Ginseng Rubra* and *Radix Ophiopogonis* preparations or for those with serious adverse reaction history.

2. Traditional Chinese medicine injections are complex in composition and unstable in nature and are prohibited for newborns, infants, pregnant women and lactating women. Patients with liver and kidney dysfunction and elderly patients should use it with caution.

3. The medicine can cause tachycardia, hypotension and other symptoms, and should be used with caution for patients with serious heart diseases.

4. *Radix Ginseng Rubra* in the prescription can improve the excitability of the body and should not be used together with cardiac glycosides and central nerve system stimulating drugs.

5. Patients with other basic diseases should use it under the

guidance of doctors.

References

[1] YIN L H, WO X D. Progress in pharmacological and clinical research of Shenmai Injection [J] . Journal of Zhejiang College of Traditional Chinese Medicine, 2011, 25 (6): 65-68.

[2] CAO X D, DING Z S, CHEN J. Pharmacological and clinical research progress of Shenmai Injection [J] . Chinese Journal of Information on Traditional Chinese Medicine, 2010, 17 (3): 104-106.

[3] WU Q S, LIU D M. Clinical application of Shenmai Injection [J] . Chinese Journal of Hospital Pharmacy, 2000, 20 (11): 676-678.

[4] LIU W H, LI C J, ZHANG J, et al. Adverse reactions of Shenmai Injection [J] . Chinese Journal of Misdiagnostics, 2011, 11 (31): 7690.

[5] YAN Z B. Analysis on the combined application and adverse reactions of Shenmai Injection [J] . World Latest Medicine Information, 2019, 19 (91): 132-133.

Qingfei Paidu Decoction

Qingfei Paidu Decoction is an innovative prescription specifically developed for the treatment of COVID-19. It is a rational and optimized combination of several classic prescriptions originated from *Treatise on Febrile Diseases* by Zhang Zhongjing mixing Shigan Decoction, Shegan Mahuang Decoction, Xiaochaihu Decoction and Wuling Powder. This medicine has been and is still being used for treating COVID-19 in several hospitals in Shanxi, Hebei, Heilongjiang and Shaanxi Provinces, China with very promising therapeutic outcomes, as manifested by efficient prevention of transition from light to severe/critical COVID-19 patients and reduction of death rate of severe/critical COVID-19 patients.

Recommended Prescription

Herba Ephedrae 9g, *Radix Glycyrrhizae Preparata* 6g, *Semen Armeniacae Amarum* 9g, raw *Gypsum Fibrosum* 15~30g (decocted first) , *Ramulus Cinnamomi* 9g, *Rhizoma Alismatis* 9g, *Polyporus Umbellatus* 9g, *Rhizoma Atractylodis Macrocephalae* 9g, *Poria* 15g, *Radix Bupleuri* 16g, *Radix Scutellariae* 6g, *Rhizoma Pinelliae Preparata* 9g, *Rhizoma Zingiberis Recens* 9g, *Radix Asteris* 9g, *Flos Farfarae* 9g, *Rhizoma Belamcandae* 9g, *Herba Asari* 6g, *Rhizoma Dioscoreae* 12g, *Fructus Aurantii Immaturus* 6g, *Pericarpium Citri Reticulatae* 6g and *Herba Pogostemonis* 9g.

Pharmacologic Effects and Mechanism

The main pharmacological effects of Maxing Shigan Decoction are relieving exterior syndrome, achieving catharsis with its cool and pungent mature, clearing lung heat and relieving asthma. Shegan Mahuang Decoction acts by ventilating lung Qi, dispelling phlegm, descending Qi and relieving cough and is suitable for symptoms such as suffocation, shortness of breath and cough of COVID-19. Wuling Powder was formulated by Zhang Zhongjing and has the effects of activating Qi and inducing diuresis. Modern pharmacological studies have proven that Xiaochaihu Decoction has antipyretic, anti-inflammatory, immune regulation, antiemetic, liver protection, gallbladder promoting and other beneficial effects. In addition, *Herba Pogostemonis* contained in Qingfei Paidu Decoction can dispel dampness, *Gypsum Fibrosum* can prevent depression and heat, and the optimized prescription can ventilate lung Qi, relieve cough, dispel cold and dampness, and protect liver and gallbladder.

Indications

Qingfei Paidu Decoction is highly recommended as a prioritized choice for treating COVID-19 in *Guidelines for the Diagnosis and Treatment of COVID-19* (Tentative 7th Edition) . Its indications include mild, common and severe patients with COVID-19. It can be used rationally in combination for the treatment of critical patients according to the actual circumstance of patients.

Dosage and Administration

Guidelines for the Diagnosis and Treatment of COVID-19 (Tentative 7th Edition) recommends the following administration methods of Qingfei Paidu Decoction:

1. Take one dose of Qingfei Paidu Decoction per day and three consecutive doses for one treatment course.

2. If conditions permit, serve half a bowl of rice soup taking the medicine each time, or one full bowl for patients with dry tongue and body fluid deficiency (rice soup can clear stomach deficiency heat and protect stomach Qi, and its Yin-nourishing effect are recorded in *Supplement to the Compendium of Materia Medica*) .

Precautions

1. Patients without fever should take a small dose of raw *Gypsum Fibrosum*, and patients with fever or high body temperature need to take a higher dose of raw *Gypsum Fibrosum* (as raw *Gypsum Fibrosum* is effective for cough and asthma due to lung heat, but it is a strong cold medicine and can readily hurt Yang Qi. Excessive dose will lead to poor appetite, listlessness, weakness, etc.) . Raw *Gypsum Fibrosum* has the function of clearing heat and purging fire. It is strictly restricted for patients with cold and typhoid cold. Pregnant women should use it with caution. Children, lactating women, the elderly and infirm, and subjects with spleen deficiency and loose stool should take it under the guidance of doctors.

2. According to the recommendation of *Guidelines for the Diagnosis and Treatment of COVID-19* (Tentative 7th Edition) , if the

symptoms are improved but the disease is not completely cured, one needs to continue to the second course of treatment. If the patient has some special conditions or other basic diseases, the prescription of the second course of treatment can be modified accordingly. Stop taking the medicine once the symptoms disappear.

3. The clinical outcomes and data from recent applications of Qingfei Paidu Decoction to patients with COVID-19 in China indicate the existence of individual differences in terms of therapeutic efficacy, and therefore the dosage of the medicine needs to be re-adjusted accordingly. Take the medicine under the guidance of doctors.

4. The prescription contains *Herba Ephedrae* which can likely cause sweating and loss of Qi. Excessive dose or long-term use of this medicine should be avoided. *Herba Ephedrae* combined with alkaloid medicines can increase toxicity and combined with cardiac glycoside can increase toxicity and induce arrhythmias.

5. The prescription contains *Radix Scutellariae* which can cause allergy. Therefore, it is restricted for those who have allergic history to any of the components in Qingfei Paidu Decoction and subjects with allergic constitution should use it with caution.

6. Patients who need to take other medicines while receiving Qingfei Paidu Decoction medication should consult a physician for appropriate solution.

References

[1] JIANG X, SUN S F, WANG Y. Research on the toxicity of ephedra [J] . Shandong Chemical Industry, 2017, 46 (14): 49-50, 54.

[2] YU Y X, TANG W, WANG J T. Discussion on the new clinical application of the classical formula Wulingsan [J] . Journal of

Traditional Chinese Medicine, 2019, 18 (06): 22-24.

[3] SUN M Y. The study on the relationship between the combination use and pharmacological effects of Xiaochaihu Decoction [D] . Beijing: Doctoral Dissertation of Beijing University of Traditional Chinese Medicine, 2003.

Prescription for Cold-dampness Stagnation in Lung Syndrome

Recommended Prescription

Raw *Herba Ephedrae* 6g, raw *Gypsum Fibrosum* 15g, *Semen Armeniacae Amarum* 9g, *Rhizoma et Radix Notopterygii* 15g, *Semen Descurainiae* 15g, *Rhizoma Dryopteris Crassirhizomae* 9g, *Lumbricus* 15g, *Radix Cynanchi Paniculati* 15g, *Herba Pogostemonis* 15g, *Herba Eupatorii* 9g, *Rhizoma Atractylodis* 15g, *Poria* 45g, raw *Rhizoma Atractylodis Macrocephalae* 30g, Jiaosanxian 27g (scorched *Fructus Hordei Germinatus* 9g, scorched *Fructus Crataegi* 9g, scorched *Massa Medicata Fermentata* 9g) , *Cortex Magnoliae Officinalis* 15g, scorched *Semen Arecae* 9g, roasted *Fructus Tsaoko* 9g and *Rhizoma Zingiberis Recens* 15g.

Pharmacologic Effects and Mechanism

The main component of *Herba Ephedrae* is ephedrine which has the effects of relieving bronchial smooth muscle spasm, diuresis, anti-inflammation and anti-virus. Combined with *Herba Ephedrae* and *Rhizoma Zingiberis Recens* can enhance perspiration, relieve cough and dispel phlegm. Combination of *Herba Ephedrae* and *Semen Armeniacae Amarum* has antitussive and antiasthmatic effects. Combination of *Herba Ephedrae*, *Rhizoma Atractylodis Macrocephalae* and *Gypsum*

Fibrosum can clear lung and relieve asthma. *Cortex Magnoliae Officinalis* contains various phenolic substances with honokiol being the main component, which primarily produce antibacterial, anti-inflammatory and muscle-relaxation effects. *Rhizoma Atractylodis* contains various volatile oils with atractylol being the main component which has sedative and smooth muscle relaxing effects. *Herba Eupatorii* contains cyme and has antibacterial, antiviral and expectorant effects. Combination of *Herba Eupatorii, Rhizoma Atractylodis* and *Cortex Magnoliae Officinalis* can be used to treat the syndrome of dampness blocking the middle energizer.

Herba Pogostemonis contains volatile oil with patchouli alcohol being the main component which can enhance digestion ability, relieve diarrhea and induce sweating. Combination of *Semen Arecae, Cortex Magnoliae Officinalis* and *Fructus Tsaoko* can be used to treat damp-heat obstruction and pivotal dereliction of duty. *Rhizoma Atractylodis* and Jiaosanxian can be combined for the treatment of dampness, invigorate spleen, Qi and stomach. *Fructus Tsaoko* contains pinene and has antitussive, expectorant, anti-inflammatory, antibacterial, digestive and diuretic effects. When combined with *Poria* (Yuling, produced from Yunnan Province) and *Semen Descurainiae* can enhance diuretic effects.

Lumbricus contains a variety of amino acids which have the effects of clearing away heat and toxic materials, relieving asthma and relieving cough. Combined of *Lumbricus* with *Herba Ephedrae* and *Semen Armeniacae Amarum* can strengthen the pharmacologic activities of clearing lung heat, eliminating phlegm, relieving cough and relieving asthma. When combined with *Rhizoma et Radix Notopterygii* and *Rhizoma Dryopteris*

Crassirhizomae, it can enhance antipyretic, analgesic and anti-viral effects. *Radix Cynanchi Paniculati* mainly contains paeonol, flavonoid glycoside and a small amount of alkaloids and has many effects such as analgesia, sedation, antibacterial, antihypertensive, blood lipid reduction, etc.

Indications

Fever, fatigue, soreness over whole body, cough, expectoration, chest tightness, suffocation, anorexia, nausea, vomiting, sticky stool and discomfort; Light tongue with tooth marks or reddish coating, white, thick and greasy fur; Soft or slippery pulse. *Guidelines for the Diagnosis and Treatment of COVID-19* (Tentative 7th Edition) recommends this prescription to patients with mild clinical manifestations mentioned above.

Dosage and Administration

Guidelines for the Diagnosis and Treatment of COVID-19 (Tentative 7th Edition) recommends that patients take 1 dose (decocting 600ml in water) by 3 times before each meal per day.

Precautions

This prescription is primarily of pungent, warm, dry and damp nature which could likely consume Qi and injure body fluid. Therefore, it should be used with caution for patients with Qi deficiency and body fluid deficiency, weak people and pregnant women. Fat can cause toxic reaction of *Rhizoma Dryopteris Crassirhizomae*, leading to headache, diarrhea and other symptoms; thus, greasy food should be avoided. Raw *Rhizoma Atractylodis Macrocephalae* is restricted for people with constipation. Patients must avoid raw, cold, greasy and spicy food while receiving medication with this prescription.

Prescription for Accumulation of Damp-heat in Lung Syndrome

Recommended Prescription

Semen Arecae 10g, *Fructus Tsaoko* 10g, *Cortex Magnoliae Officinalis* 10g, *Rhizoma Anemarrhenae* 10g, *Radix Scutellariae* 10g, *Radix Bupleuri* 10g, *Radix Paeoniae Rubra* 10g, *Fructus Forsythiae* 15g, *Herba Artemisiae Annuae* 10g (after other medicines), *Rhizoma Atractylodis* 10g, *Folium Isatidis* 10g and raw *Radix Glycyrrhizae* 5g.

Pharmacologic Effects and Mechanism

Fructus Forsythiae contains triterpene saponins which have broad-spectrum antibacterial, antiviral, antipyretic, antihypertensive effects. *Radix Glycyrrhizae* contains triterpenes which have the effects of eliminating phlegm, relieving asthma, resisting bacteria, virus and inflammation, etc. , and can be combined with *Fructus Forsythiae* to enhance the effects of clearing away heat and toxic materials. *Radix Scutellariae* contains baicalein which has antipyretic, antihypertensive, sedative, antibacterial, antiviral effects. *Radix Bupleuri* contains saikosaponin and a variety of volatile oil components which can produce inhibitory effects on central nerve system such as sedation, analgesia, antipyretic, antitussive, etc. It can be used together with *Radix Scutellariae* to enhance the effects of clearing heat and relieving exterior syndrome and treating fever and headache. *Herba Artemisiae Annuae* contains sesquiterpenes, flavonoids, coumarins and other components and has anti-malaria, antipyretic and analgesic, antibacterial and antiviral effects. It can be combined with *Radix Scutellariae* to enhance its antiviral, antipyretic and analgesic effects. *Rhizoma Atractylodis* contains a variety of volatile oils with atractylol being the main component which has sedative effects on the central nerve system and can relax smooth muscle.

Fructus Tsaoko contains pinene and has antitussive, expectorant, anti-inflammatory, antibacterial, digestive and diuretic effects. *Semen Arecae* contains arecoline which mainly elicit anthelmintic and antiviral effects and can promote digestion. It can be used together with *Fructus Tsaoko* to enhance the antibacterial, antiviral and anthelmintic effects.

Cortex Magnoliae Officinalis contains honokiol and has antibacterial, anti-inflammatory and central muscle relaxation effects. *Radix Paeoniae Rubra* contains paeoniflorin and other components and has sedative, anti-inflammatory, analgesic, antipyretic and anticonvulsant effects. It can be combined with *Radix Scutellariae* to enhance its heat-clearing and detoxifying effects. *Folium Isatidis* contains a variety of amino acids, indirubin B and other components and has antibacterial, antiviral, heat-clearing and detoxifying effects. *Rhizoma Anemarrhenae* contains anemarrhena saponins and other components and has antipyretic, antibacterial and antiviral effects.

Indications

Low fever or no fever, slight aversion to cold, fatigue, heavy head and body drowsiness, muscle soreness, dry cough and less expectoration, sore throat, dry mouth and no desire to drink, chest tightness and epigastric fullness, no sweat or unsmooth sweating, vomiting, anorexia, and loose or sticky stool; Reddish tongue, white, thick, greasy or thin and yellow coating. Slippery or soft pulse. *Guidelines for the Diagnosis and Treatment of COVID-19* (Tentative 7th Edition) recommends this prescription for patients with mild clinical manifestations mentioned above.

Dosage and Administration

Guidelines for the Diagnosis and Treatment of COVID-19 (Tentative 7th Edition) recommends 1 dose (400ml decocted in water) per day, divided into two equal-volume serves with one taken in the morning and the second one in the evening.

Precautions

Most of the prescription are of bitter cold, heat-clearing and exterior-relieving medicines, which can likely hurt the stomach and spleen. Therefore, those with spleen and stomach deficiency cold, weak people and pregnant women should use the medicine with caution. *Radix Glycyrrhizae* should not be used along with *Radix Euphorbiae Pekinensis*, *Flos Genkwa*, *Radix Euphorbiae Kansui* and *Sargassum*. *Radix Paeoniae Rubra* is not compatible with *Veratri Nigri Radix et Rhizoma* and thus, they cannot be used together. Patients in medication with this prescription must avoid raw, cold, greasy and spicy food.

References

[1] MIAO L, QI C. On the syndrome of Mahuang almond Liquorice Plaster Decoction [J]. Journal of Heze Medical College, 2011, 23 (04): 46-47.

[2] HU F Y, FAN Y H, FAN X S, et al. Effect of Houpu Mahuangtang on airway inflammation and expression of TRPA1, TRPV1 mRNA and protein in asthmatic mice [J]. Chinese Journal of Experimental Traditional Medical Formulae, 2020, 26 (01): 37-42.

[3] WANG D M, WANG Y Y, MU Y J, et al. Feasibility analysis on the treatment of haze inhalation lung injury with Fuling, almond and Liquorice Decoction [J]. Hebei Journal of Traditional Chinese Medicine, 2019, 41 (05): 771-774.

[4] JIANG W, XUE Q, LI J, et al. The clinical effect of Mahuang forsythia and red bean Decoction on damp and hot cough [J] . Medical & Pharmaceutical Journal of Chinese People's Liberation Army, 2019, 31 (10): 85-88.

Prescription for Stagnation of Damp Toxicity in Lung Syndrome

Recommended Prescription

Raw *Herba Ephedrae* 6g, *Semen Armeniacae Amarum* 15g, raw *Gypsum Fibrosum* 30g, raw *Semen Coicis* 30g, *Rhizoma Areactylodis Lanceae* 10g, *Herba Pogostemonis* 15g, *Herba Artemisiae Annuae* 12g, *Rhizoma Polygoni Cuspidati* 20g, *Herba Verbenae* 30g, dry *Rhizoma Phragmitis* 30g, *Semen Descurainiae* 15g, *Exocarpium Citri Grandis* 15g and raw *Radix Glycyrrhizae* 10g.

Pharmacologic Effects and Mechanism

The main active ingredients of raw *Herba Ephedrae* are ephedrine and feruloylhistamine which have analgesic, antibacterial, antiviral, anti-inflammatory, antipyretic, antihypertensive, diuretic and antiasthmatic effects. The main active ingredients of *Semen Armeniacae Amarum* are amygdalin, fatty oil, and amygdalase which have the effects of relieving cough and asthma, resisting inflammation and pain, resisting oxidation, relaxing bowels, reducing blood lipid, and regulating immune function. Raw *Gypsum Fibrosum* has antipyretic, analgesic and immunity-improving activities.

The main active ingredients of raw *Semen Coicis* are coixenolide seed ester and fatty acid, which have the effects of lowering blood lipid, resisting inflammation and relieving pain, and improving immunity. The main active ingredients of *Rhizoma Areactylodis Lanceae* are atractylodin and hinesol which have the effects of relieving intestinal spasm, protecting gastric mucosa and resisting bacteria. The main active ingredients of *Herba Pogostemonis* are pogostone, and β-caryophyllene which have antiviral, antibacterial, antifungal, digestion-promoting, anti-inflammatory, analgesic and antipyretic effects. The main active ingredient of *Herba Artemisiae Annuae* is artemisinin which has antimalarial, antibacterial, antiviral and antiarrhythmic effects.

The main active ingredients of *Rhizoma Polygoni Cuspidati* are anthraquinone compounds which have antibacterial, antitussive, antiasthmatic, antihypertensive, antiviral, antitumor, sedative and microcirculation-improving effects. The main active ingredient of *Herba Verbenae* is verbenalin which can exert anti-inflammatory, analgesic, antitussive, antimalarial and antibacterial effects. The main chemical composition of dry *Rhizoma Phragmitis* is polysaccharide which has liver protection and antibacterial effects. The main active ingredient of *Semen Descurainiae* is sinigrin which has antitussive, antiasthmatic, cardiotonic and antibacterial effects. The main active ingredient of *Exocarpium Citri Grandis* is citral which has sedative, antimicrobial, antitussive and expectorant effects. The main active ingredient of raw *Radix Glycyrrhizae* is glycyrrhizin which has antibacterial, antiviral, anti-inflammatory, antitussive, spasmolytic and antiallergic effects.

Indications

This prescription is mainly used for the syndrome of stagnation of damp-toxicity in lung. It is recommended for patients with common COVID-19 in *Guidelines for the Diagnosis and Treatment of COVID-19* (Tentative 7th Edition) . Its clinical manifestations are fever, cough, less phlegm, or yellow phlegm, suffocation, shortness of breath, abdominal distension and constipation, dark red tongue, fat tongue body, yellow and greasy or yellow and dry tongue coating, and slippery and fast or stringy pulse.

Dosage and Administration

Guidelines for the Diagnosis and Treatment of COVID-19 (Tentative 7th Edition) recommends 1 dose (400ml preparation by after decocted in water) per day, separated into two equal-volume parts with one taken in the morning and the second one in the evening.

Precautions

1. The prescription contains raw *Herba Ephedrae*, and is forbidden for people with body deficiency, spontaneous sweat, night sweat and deficient dyspnea.

2. The prescription contains raw *Semen Coicis* and must be used with caution for patients with spleen constipation, pregnant women, and patients with stomach deficiency.

3. The prescription contains *Herba Artemisiae Annuae* and must not be used for patients with diarrhea or dietary stagnation and diarrhea caused by postpartum blood deficiency and internal cold.

4. The prescription contains *Radix Glycyrrhizae* which can exert inhibitory effects on central nervous system, and thus infants and elderly patients must not be in overdose for a long time. In addition, *Radix Glycyrrhizae* can exaggerate hypertension, and thus hypertensive patients must not take large quantities for a long time. Patients with acute nephritis or aldosteronism and hypokalemia must not take this medicine.

Prescription for Cold-dampness Obstructing Lung Syndrome

Recommended Prescription

Rhizoma Atractylodis 15g, *Pericarpium Citri Reticulatae* 10g, *Cortex Magnoliae Officinalis* 10g, *Herba Pogostemonis* 10g, *Fructus Tsaoko* 6g, raw *Herba Ephedrae* 6g, *Rhizoma et Radix Notopterygii* 10g, *Rhizoma Zingiberis Recens* 10g and *Semen Arecae* 10g.

Pharmacologic Effects and Mechanism

The main active ingredients of *Rhizoma Atractylodis* are atractylol, hinesol, and β-cineole which have significant inhibitory effects on *Mycobacterium tuberculosis*, *Staphylococcus aureus*, *Escherichia coli* and *Pseudomonas aeruginosa*, and have anti-inflammatory, digestion and absorption-promoting and immune-regulating effects. *Pericarpium Citri Reticulatae* has pharmacological activities of protecting heart, eliminating phlegm, relieving asthma, swelling and vomiting. *Cortex Magnoliae Officinalis* decoction has inhibitory effects on pneumococcus, *Diphtheria bacillus*, hemolytic streptococcus, *Staphylococcus aureus* and various skin fungi.

The volatile oil of *Herba Pogostemonis* can promote gastric juice secretion, enhance digestion ability, relieve spasm on gastrointestinal tract, and has antibacterial, antidiarrheal, microvascularization and other effects. The main active ingredient 1, 8-cineole in *Fructus Tsaoko* has antitussive, expectorant, analgesic, antipyretic, antiasthmatic, antibacterial and anti-inflammatory effects. The main active ingredient of raw *Herba Ephedrae* is ephedrine which has analgesic, antibacterial, antiviral, anti-inflammatory, antipyretic, antihypertensive, diuresis and antiasthmatic effects. The main active ingredient of *Rhizoma et Radix Notopterygii* is coumarin extract compound which has antipyretic, analgesic, anti-inflammatory and antiarrhythmic effects.

The main active ingredients of *Rhizoma Zingiberis Recens* are gingerol, and zingiberene which have obvious inhibitory effects on *Staphylococcus aureus*, *Staphylococcus albus*, *Typhoid bacillus*, *Shigella sonnei* and *Pseudomonas aeruginosa*. In addition, *Rhizoma Zingiberis Recens* also has antiplatelet aggregation, respiratory system excitation, sedation and antioxidation effects. *Semen Arecae* can promote digestion and absorption and resist pathogenic microorganisms.

Indications

This prescription is mainly used for treating cold-dampness obstruction of lung syndrome. *Guidelines for the Diagnosis and Treatment of COVID-19* (Tentative 7th Edition) recommends it for COVID-19 patients with clinical manifestations including low fever, body heat not rising, or not hot, dry cough, less phlegm, tiredness and fatigue, chest tightness, epigastric fullness, or vomiting and aversion, loose stool, pale or reddish tongue, white or greasy tongue coating, and soft pulse.

Dosage and Administration

Guidelines for the Diagnosis and Treatment of COVID-19 (Tentative 7th Edition) recommends 1 dose per day by preparing 400ml decoction in water and separating into two equal-volume parts, with the first one taken in the morning and the second one in the evening.

Precautions

1. The prescription contains *Rhizoma Atractylodis* which must

not be used for people with Yin deficiency, internal heat and Qi deficiency and hyperhidrosis.

2. The prescription contains *Cortex Magnoliae Officinalis* and is not suitable for pregnant women.

3. The prescription contains raw *Herba Ephedrae* and is forbidden for people with body deficiency, spontaneous sweat, night sweat and deficient dyspnea.

References

ZHANG M F, SHEN Y Q. Research advances on difference of pharmacologic effects of Atractylodis Rhizoma before and after processing [J] . Anti-Infection Pharmacy, 2017, 14 (03): 481-485.

Prescription for Epidemic Toxin Blocking Lung Syndrome

Recommended Prescription

Raw *Herba Ephedrae* 6g, *Semen Armeniacae Amarum* 9g, raw *Gypsum Fibrosum* 15g, *Radix Glycyrrhizae* 3g, *Herba Pogostemonis* 10g (after other medicines) , *Cortex Magnoliae Officinalis* 10g, *Rhizoma Atractylodis* 15g, *Fructus Tsaoko* 10g, *Rhizoma Pinelliae Preparatum* 9g, *Poria* 15g, raw *Radix et Rhizoma Rhei* 5g (after other medicines) , raw *Radix Astragali seu Hedysari* 10g, *Semen Descurainiae* 10g and *Radix Paeoniae Rubra* 10g.

Pharmacologic Effects and Mechanism

The main active ingredient of raw *Herba Ephedrae* is ephedrine which has analgesic, antibacterial, antiviral, anti-inflammatory, antipyretic, antihypertensive, diuresis and antiasthmatic effects. The main active ingredients of *Semen Armeniacae Amarum* are amygdalin, fatty oil, and amygdalase which act by relieving cough and asthma, resisting inflammation and pain, resisting oxidation, relaxing bowels, reducing blood lipid, and regulating immune function. Raw *Gypsum Fibrosum* has antipyretic, analgesic and immunity-improving effects.

The main active ingredient of *Radix Glycyrrhizae* is glycyrrhizin which has antibacterial, antiviral, anti-inflammatory, antitussive, spasmolytic and antiallergic effects. The volatile oil of *Herba Pogostemonis* can promote gastric juice secretion, enhance digestion, relieve spasm on gastrointestinal tract, and exert antibacterial, antidiarrheal, microvascularization dilation and other effects. *Cortex Magnoliae Officinalis* decoction has inhibitory effects on pneumococcus, *Diphtheria bacillus*, hemolytic streptococcus, *Staphylococcus aureus* and various skin fungi. The main active ingredients of *Rhizoma Atractylodis* are atractylodin and hinesol which have the effects of relieving intestinal spasm, protecting gastric mucosa and resisting bacteria. The main active ingredient of *Fructus Tsaoko* is 1, 8-cineole which has antitussive, expectorant, analgesic, antipyretic, antiasthmatic, antibacterial and anti-inflammatory effects.

Rhizoma Pinelliae Preparatum is a processed product of *Rhizoma Pinelliae*. Its main active ingredient is 3-acetylamino-5-methylisazole and can elicit antitussive, antiemetic, antiarrhythmic, antihypertensive and coagulant effects. The main active ingredient of *Poria* is β-poria polysaccharide which has diuresis and antibacterial effects. The main active ingredients of raw *Radix et Rhizoma Rhei* are rhein, emodin, and aloe-emodin which have the effects of promoting digestion, resisting bacteria, reducing blood lipid, relieving bronchospasm and promoting blood coagulation. The main active ingredient of raw *Radix Astragali seu Hedysari* is astragaloside, which has the effects of improving immunity, resisting bacteria, resisting viruses and inducing diuresis. The main active ingredient of *Semen Descurainiae* is sinigrin which has antitussive, antiasthmatic, cardiotonic and antibacterial effects. The main active ingredient of *Radix Paeoniae Rubra* is paeoniflorin which has anti-platelet aggregation, antithrombosis and liver protection effects.

Indications

This prescription is mainly used for treating lung obstruction due to epidemic toxin. *Guidelines for the Diagnosis and Treatment of COVID-19* (Tentative 7th Edition) recommends it for severe COVID-19 patients with clinical manifestations including fever, red face, cough, yellow and sticky phlegm, or bloody phlegm, dyspnea, fatigue and tiredness, dry, bitter and sticky mouth, nausea and anorexia, poor stool, short and red urine, red tongue, yellow and greasy tongue coating, and slippery and fast pulse.

Dosage and Administration

Guidelines for the Diagnosis and Treatment of COVID-19 (Tentative 7th Edition) recommends 1~2 doses per day by oral or nasal feeding in the form of decoction prepared with water, which are to be separated into 2~4 portions in 100~200ml each and served separately in a day.

Precautions

1. The prescription contains raw *Herba Ephedrae* and is forbidden for people with body deficiency, spontaneous sweat, night sweat and deficient dyspnea.

2. The prescription contains *Cortex Magnoliae Officinalis* and is not suitable for pregnant women.

3. The prescription contains *Rhizoma Pinelliae Preparatum*

and must not be combined with aconitum medicines. It should not be taken by subjects with any of the blood syndromes, Yin deficiency, dryness, cough, body fluid injury and thirst.

Prescription for Syndrome of Blazing Heat in Both Qi and Nutrient Phases

Recommended Prescription

Raw *Gypsum Fibrosum* 30~60g (decocted first) , *Rhizoma Anemarrhenae* 30g, *Radix Rehmanniae Recens* 30~60g, *Cornu Bubali* 30g (decocted first) , *Radix Paeoniae Rubra* 30g, *Radix Scrophulariae* 30g, *Fructus Forsythiae* 15g, *Cortex Moutan Radicis* 15g, *Rhizoma Coptidis* 6g, *Herba Lophatheri* 12g, *Semen Descurainiae* 15g and raw *Radix Glycyrrhizae* 6g.

Pharmacologic Effects and Mechanism

Raw *Gypsum Fibrosum* has antipyretic, analgesic and immunity-improving effects. The main active ingredients of *Rhizoma Anemarrhenae* are timosaponin and other saponins which have antibacterial and adrenocorticotropic hormone secretion effects. The water extraction of *Radix Rehmanniae Recens* can exert actions by resisting pulmonary fibrosis, promoting hematopoiesis, resisting inflammation, improving glycolipid metabolism and protecting gastric mucosa.

The main active components of *Cornu Bubali* are cholesterol and various amino acids which have cardiotonic, sedative and anticonvulsant effects. The main active ingredient of *Radix Paeoniae Rubra* is paeoniflorin which has anti-platelet aggregation, antithrombosis and liver protection effects. *Radix Scrophulariae* has antibacterial, antifungal, sedative, antihypertensive, cardiotonic, vasodilator and anticonvulsant effects. The main active ingredients of *Fructus Forsythiae* are forsythia phenol and forsythin which have antibacterial, antiemetic, cardiotonic and diuretic effects. The main active ingredient of *Cortex Moutan Radicis* is paeonol which has antibacterial, sedative, hypnotic, analgesic and antihypertensive effects.

The main component of *Rhizoma Coptidis* is berberine which has antibacterial, antiarrhythmic, antidiarrheal and anti-inflammatory effects. The main active components of *Herba Lophatheri* are polysaccharides and flavonoids which have antioxidant, anti-myocardial ischemia, vasoconstriction, bacteriostasis and liver injury protection effects. The main active ingredient of *Semen Descurainiae* is sinigrin which has antitussive, antiasthmatic, cardiotonic and antibacterial effects. The main active ingredient of raw *Radix Glycyrrhizae* is glycyrrhizin which has antibacterial, antiviral, anti-inflammatory, antitussive, spasmolytic and antiallergic effects.

Indications

This prescription is mainly used for treating Syndrome of Blazing Heat in Both Qi and Nutrient Phases. It is recommended for patients with severe COVID-19 in *Guidelines for the Diagnosis and Treatment of COVID-19* (Tentative 7th Edition) . Its clinical manifestations include hot polydipsia, dyspnea, delirium, dizziness, wrong vision, macula, vomiting blood, epistaxis, limb convulsions, crimson tongue with little or no coating, heavy, thin and fast pulse, or floating and fast pulse.

Dosage and Administration

Guidelines for the Diagnosis and Treatment of COVID-19 (Tentative 7th Edition) recommends 1 dose in 2~4 times per day via oral or nasal administration, 100~200ml each time with the medicine decocted with water (decocting *Gypsum Fibrosum* and *Cornu Bubali* first followed by other ingredients).

Precautions

1. The prescription contains *Cornu Bubali*. People with middle deficiency and cold stomach should take it with caution. A large dose often causes upper abdominal discomfort, nausea, abdominal distension, loss of appetite and other reactions.

2. The prescription contains *Radix Paeoniae Rubra*. Patients with blood deficiency and carbuncle with broken abscess should use it with caution.

3. The prescription contains *Radix Scrophulariae* and should not be taken along with *Veratri Nigri Radix et Rhizoma*. It is forbidden for people with dampness in spleen, loose stool caused by spleen deficiency.

4. The prescription contains *Fructus Forsythiae* and is forbidden for patients with spleen and stomach deficiency, Qi deficiency and fever, broken abscess, and pale pus.

5. The prescription contains *Cortex Moutan Radicis*. Patients with blood deficiency and cold, pregnant women and patients with menorrhagia should use it with caution.

6. The prescription contains *Rhizoma Coptidis*, which is of severe cold nature. Excessive and long-term administration can readily damage the spleen and stomach. Patients with deficiency and cold in the spleen and stomach must not take this medicine. In addition, *Rhizoma Coptidis* is bitter and dry, which can damage Yin and fluid, and thus it should be used with caution for people with Yin deficiency and fluid injury.

7. The prescription contains *Radix Glycyrrhizae* which can

negatively affect central nervous system, and infants and elderly patients therefore must not take it in large quantities for a long time. In addition, *Radix Glycyrrhizae* can exaggerate hypertension and hypertensive patients must not take it in large quantities for a long time. Patients with acute nephritis, aldosteronism or hypokalemia should not use it.

References

LIANG D, CHEN Q L, CHEN Q X. Research progress in pharmacological action of bamboo leaves [J] . Journal of clinical rational drug use, 2014, 7 (11): 89-90.

Prescription for Syndrome of Internal Blockade and External Collapse

Recommended Prescription

Radix Ginseng 15g, *Radix Aconiti Lateralis Preparata* tablet (Heishun tablet) 10g (decocted first) , and *Fructus Corni* 15g, along with Suhexiang Pill or Angong Niuhuang Pill.

(1) Angong Niuhuang Pill contains *Calculus Bovis, Cornu Bubali* Concentrated Powder, Artificial *Moschus, Margarita, Cinnabaris, Realgar, Rhizoma Coptidis, Radix Scutellariae, Fructus Gardeniae, Radix Curcumae,* and *Borneolum Syntheticum.*

(2) Suhexiang Pill contains *Styrax, Benzoinum, Borneolum Syntheticum, Cornu Bubali* Concentrated Powder, Artificial *Moschus, Lignum Santali Albi, Lignum Aquilariae Resinatum, Flos Caryophylli, Rhizoma Cyperi, Radix Aucklandiae, Olibanum* (pre-

pared) , *Fructus Piperis Longi, Rhizoma Atractylodis Macrocephalae, Fructus Chebulae* flesh, and *Cinnabaris*.

Pharmacologic Effects and Mechanism

Radix Ginseng restores pulse for relieving desertion, promotes fluid production and tranquilizes mind. *Heishun* Tablet replenishes spleen and Yang, dispels cold and relieves pain. It has similar effects to *Radix Ginseng*, being both good medicines for "returning Yang and saving inverse". *Fructus Corni* stimulates fluid production to quench thirst and astringes spermatorrhea for relieving desertion. Angong Niuhuang Pill, a classic aid prescription in traditional Chinese medicine, is a compound medicine originated from Wu Jutong's *Detailed Analysis of Epidemic Warm Diseases* in Qing Dynasty. Together with Zixue Pill and Zhibao Pill, it is known as one of the "three treasure cold formulas for resuscitation for warm disease in traditional Chinese medicine", which acts by clearing away heat and toxic materials, relieving convulsion and inducing resuscitation. Suhexiang Pill is a famous medicine for warming, dredging and inducing resuscitation, which can induce resuscitation with fragrance, promote Qi circulation and relieve pain.

Studies have shown that ginsenoside, the main component of *Radix Ginseng*, has many beneficial effects, such as anti-inflammation, anti-oxidation, anti-aging and cardiovascular protection. Aconitine, the main component of *Heishun* Tablet, has obvious effects of strengthening heart, resisting inflammation, analgesia, etc. Polysaccharides, organic acids and iridoid substances contained in *Fructus Corni* can also exert anti-inflammatory, analgesic, cardiotonic, endocrine regulating effects.

Berberine and baicalin contained in *Rhizoma Coptidis* and *Radix Scutellariae* in the combination of Angong Niuhuang Pill produce pharmacological effects by clearing away heat and purging fire and decreasing fever caused by bacterial toxins. *Calculus Bovis* and *Cinnabaris* inhibit the excitability of the central nervous system and have sedative, hypnotic and anticonvulsant effects. Muscone contained in *Moschus* can improve the function of central nervous system and reduce cerebral ischemic and hypoxic injuries. *Borneolum Syntheticum* contains D-borneol and has inhibitory effects on *Escherichia coli* and *Staphylococcus aureus*. Combination of *Margarita* powder and *Calculus Bovis* inhibit fungal infection.

Suhexiang Pill, a compound medicine, has various pharmacologic effects such as anti-inflammatory, cardiovascular protection, neurological function protection, etc. *Styrax*, the main component, can inhibit platelet aggregation, tolerate myocardial ischemia, weaken vasoconstriction, resist oxidative stress, etc. It can reduce myocardial ischemia injury and protect myocardial cells. The lipid-soluble volatile components contained in *Styrax* enable it to penetrate the blood-brain barrier, reduce free radical damage and inflammatory reaction of nerve cells, protect nerve cells from damages induced by ischemia and hypoxia, and reduce cerebral ischemia-reperfusion injury. Cinnamic acid, an effective component of *Styrax*, has the effects of bacteriostasis, antisepsis, antidiarrhea and leukocyte increase, and can relieve local inflammation.

Indications

Radix Ginseng, Radix Aconiti Lateralis Preparata Tablet and *Fructus Corni* can be used together to treat lung deficiency, asthma and cough, shortness of breath and asthma, collapse of Yang, and cold limb and slight pulse by correcting deficiency of Qi, blood and body fluid. Combined with Angong Niuhuang Pill, they can be used for high fever convulsion and delirium caused by encephalitis, meningitis, toxic encephalopathy, cerebral hemorrhage, septicemia and cerebral apoplexy. Combined with Suhexiang Pill, they can be used for phlegm coma, apoplexy hemiplegia, and convulsion caused by phlegm obstruction of the heart and orifices. The prescription can be used for fever caused by upper respiratory tract infection, pneumonia, acute tonsillitis, and acute enteritis to effectively improve asthma and abdominal distension symptoms. It can also be used for fever, headache, convulsion and consciousness disorder caused by viral encephalitis. Combined with western medicine, it can be used to treat pulmonary encephalopathy with "phlegm turbidity obscuring heart" as the main syndrome, as well as an adjuvant treatment of acute severe craniocerebral injury, cerebral arteriosclerosis, stroke and angina pectoris. *Guidelines for the Diagnosis and Treatment of COVID-19* (Tentative 7th Edition) recommends this prescription for critical COVID-19 patients with internal closure and external collapse to relieve the symptoms of dyspnea, asthma, faintness, dysphoria, sweating and cold limbs.

Dosage and Administration

Guidelines for the Diagnosis and Treatment of COVID-19 (Tentative 7th Edition) recommends the prescription for severe COVID-19 patients with the following directions: Ginseng 15g, Heishun tablet 10g (decocting first) , Cornus 15g, and Suhexiang Pill or Angong Niuhuang Pill. Angong Niuhuang Pill and Suhexiang Pill are both Chinese patent medicines. Dosage forms are different depending on different pharmaceuticals, and to choose the right one for a right person with right symptoms, consult the drug manual beforehand.

Precautions

1. **Allergic reactions** Patients who use the prescription in

large quantities at a single time are prone to allergic reactions, mainly manifested as rash and urticaria, and anaphylactic shock in severe
cases.

2. Respiratory and digestive system injury   Angong
Niuhuang Pill in the prescription can likely cause dyspnea, nausea, vomiting, diarrhea and other symptoms.

3. Angong Niuhuang Pill in the prescription contains *Realgar*, the main component of which is arsenic sulfide. Arsenic poisoning can occur after long-term application, which is manifested as
skin damage, such as dry skin, papules, herpes, exfoliative dermatitis, pigmentation, etc. It should not be combined with nitrite, ferrous
salt, nitrate and sulfate medicines to avoid weakening of curative effects or strengthening of toxicity. It should not be used with enzyme
medicines to avoid forming insoluble precipitates and inhibiting
enzyme activity.

4. Mercury poisoning   Both Angong Niuhuang Pill and
Suhexiang Pill in the prescription contain *Cinnabaris*, the main component of which is mercury sulfide. Long-term application can cause
neurotoxicity, liver and kidney toxicity, reproductive toxicity, coma
and even death due to acute poisoning.

5. *Radix Ginseng* in the prescription can improve the excitability of the body and should not be used together with cardiac glycosides and central stimulating medicines to avoid poisoning. Ginsenoside is easy to hydrolyze and loses its pharmacologic activities in
acidic environment, and thus must not be combined with medicines
with strong acidity. Ginsenoside combined with metal-containing
salt medicines are likely to form precipitates, and thus they should
not be taken together.

6. The prescription contains *Radix Ginseng* and Heishun

tablet. *Radix Aconiti Lateralis Preparata* tablets are one of the processed products of *Radix Aconiti Lateralis Preparata*. According to the incompatibility guide of traditional Chinese medicine, the prescription should not be used with *Veratri Nigri Radix et Rhizoma, Faeces Togopteri, Rhizoma Pinelliae, Fructus Trichosanthis, Bulbus Fritillaria, Radix Ampelopsis, Rhizoma Bletillae*, and some other medicines as well.

7. It is not suitable to be combined with hormone medicines for a long time in case of kidney Yin deficiency and aggravate Yin essence loss in the body.

8. The prescription should not be taken together with berberine, to retain the full antibacterial efficacy of the latter.

9. The medical property of this prescription is fierce, and the dosage and course of treatment should be put under strict control for medication. Overdose of this prescription must be strictly avoided.

10. Patients with liver and kidney dysfunction, the elderly, children and pregnant women should not take the prescription.

11. Patients complicated with other basic diseases should take it under the guidance of doctors.

References

[1] LI D, LI X M, ZHOU N. Pharmacological action and clinical application of Angong Niuhuang Pill [J]. Journal of Navy Medicine, 2007, 28 (2): 179-181.

[2] WANG Y, XU Z P, WANG J, et al. Summary of Storax [J]. Pharmacy and Clinics of Chinese Materia Medica, 2013, 4 (3): 49-51.

[3] BIAN J, ZHANG H Y. Study on ancient and modern application of Suhexiang Pill [J]. Clinical Journal of Traditional Chinese Medicine, 2016, 28 (6): 875-878.

[4] CHEN L Y, YU R, MA J Y, et al. Clinical Adverse Reaction of Realgar [J] . Chinese Journal of Information on Traditional Chinese Medicine, 2018, 35 (6): 17-20.

[5] DING T, LUO J Y, HAN X, et al. Advances of toxicity evaluation of cinnabar and compatibility necessity analysis [J] . China Journal of Chinese Materia Medica, 2016, 41 (24): 4533-4540.

[6] SHAN M, WEI F J. Incompatibility between cinnabar and bromides [J] . Journal of Hebei Medical College for Continuing Education, 2001, 18 (1): 46.

[7] TANG J Y, LI S J, WANG Y, et al. Research progress on chemical components and pharmacological effects of *Oplopanax elatus* [J] . Chinese Traditional Patent Medicine, 2020, 42 (1): 156-161.

[8] YUAN W. Pharmacological study on aconite [J] . Clinical Journal of Chinese Medicine, 2018, 10 (4): 145-147.

[9] ZHOU Y C, ZHANG L J, ZHANG Y L. New progress in the study of chemical constituents and pharmacological action of Cornus officinalis [J] . Chinese Journal of Information on Traditional Chinese Medicine, 2020, 37 (1): 114-120.

Prescription for Syndrome of Qi Deficiency of Lung and Spleen

Recommended Prescription

Rhizoma Pinelliae Preparatum 9g, *Pericarpium Citri Reticulatae* 10g, *Radix Codonopsis* 15g, roasted *Radix Astragali seu Hedysari* 30g, stir-fried *Rhizoma Atractylodis Macrocephalae* 10g, *Poria* 15g, *Herba Pogostemonis* 10g, *Fructus Amomi Villosi* 6g (after other medicines) and *Radix Glycyrrhizae* 6g.

Pharmacologic Effects and Mechanism

This prescription is a revised version of Liujunzi Decoction. Liujunzi Decoction is mainly composed of *Radix Ginseng, Rhizoma Atractylodis Macrocephalae, Poria, Radix Glycyrrhizae, Pericarpium Citri Reticulatae*, and *Rhizoma Pinelliae* and it has the effects of invigorating Qi, invigorating spleen, and eliminating dampness and phlegm. Of the multiple ingredients, *Rhizoma Pinelliae* and *Pericarpium Citri Reticulatae* have pharmacological activities of eliminating dampness and phlegm and relieving asthma and vomiting. *Rhizoma Atractylodis Macrocephalae* and *Radix Ginseng* act by invigorating Qi and spleen and eliminating dampness and diuresis. *Poria* and *Radix Glycyrrhizae* have the effects of invigorating Qi, harmonizing middle warmer, regulating spleen, and eliminating dampness and phlegm. The above-described medicines cooperate to confer the ability of reducing inflammatory cell infiltration, inhibiting gastric acid secretion and gastric mucosal lesions, and improving immune function.

This prescription can be blended with roasted *Radix Astragali seu Hedysari, Herba Pogostemonis* and *Fructus Amomi Villosi*. Of the additions, *Radix Astragali seu Hedysari* has the effects of invigorating Qi and Yang, diuresis and detoxification, and consolidating exterior and stopping perspiration and can therefore enhance immunity, reduce blood pressure, protect cardiovascular system, regulate blood sugar, inhibit virus, etc. *Herba Pogostemonis* can regulate gastrointestinal function and has antibacterial, antiviral, anti-inflammatory, analgesic and antipyretic effects. *Fructus Amomi Villosi* can dispel dampness, stop vomiting, reduce Qi and expectoration, relieve alcohol, promote intestinal peristalsis and inhibit platelet aggregation.

Indications

The prescription is suitable for patients with shortness of breath, tiredness, fatigue, anorexia, vomiting, fullness, weak stool, loose stool, pale and fat tongue, and white and greasy tongue coating. *Guidelines for the Diagnosis and Treatment of COVID-19* (Tentative 7th Edition) recommends this prescription for patients in the recovery period.

Dosage and Administration

Guidelines for the Diagnosis and Treatment of COVID-19 (Tentative 7th Edition) recommend to take 1 dose per day, decocted 400ml in water, and take it twice with one in the morning and the other in the evening.

Precautions

1. Patients in medication with this prescription should pay attention to avoiding raw, cold, greasy and spicy food.

2. *Rhizoma Pinelliae Preparatum* can reduce the anti-inflammatory activity of aconitum and is not suitable to be used together with the latter.

3. *Radix Astragali seu Hedysari* has the effects of helping heat and supplementing fire and is restricted for patients with damp heat or allergy.

4. *Fructus Amomi Villosi* can likely cause allergic reactions, which are manifested as rashes or lumps in abdomen and genitals. If allergic reactions occur, the medication must be ceased immediately.

References

[1] SUN L, DAI Y F, LU X Q, et al. Screening and exploring the key targets and potential diseases of Liujunzi Decoction based on systems pharmacology [J] . Global Chinese Medicine, 2018, 11 (02): 62-68.

[2] ZHANG G Y. Chinese medicine Huangqi pharmacological functions and clinical application research [J] . Practical Journal of Cardiac

Cerebral Pneumal and Vascular Disease, 2012, 20 (06): 135-136.

[3] REN S Z, JIN D J, ZHANG J Q, et al. Research progress in pharmacological action of Pogostemon cablin [J]. Modern Chinese Medicine, 2006, 8 (8): 27-29.

[4] KE B, SHI L. Exploring clinical efficacy of *Fructus Amomi* [J]. China Journal of Traditional Chinese Medicine and Pharmacy, 2012, 27 (01): 132-133.

[5] LAI Z Z, ZHANG L, LI Y, et al. Research of weaken anti-inflammatory effects and reduced characterization on Pinelliae Rhizoma and Aconiti Kusnezoffii Radix [J]. Chinese Journal of Experimental Traditional Medical Formulae, 2015, 21 (17): 84-87.

Prescription for Syndrome of Deficiency of both Qi and Yin

Recommended Prescription

Radix Adenophorae 10g, *Radix Glehniae* 10g, *Radix Ophiopogonis* 15g, *Radix Panacis Quinquefolii* 6g, *Fructus Schisandrae Chinensis* 6g, raw *Gypsum Fibrosum* 15g, *Herba Lophatheri* 10g, *Folium Mori* 10g, *Rhizoma Phragmitis* 15g, *Radix Salviae Miltiorrhizae* 15g and raw *Radix Glycyrrhizae* 6g.

Pharmacologic Effects and Mechanism

This prescription is formulated based on Zhuye Shigao Decoction which possesses the properties of clearing heat, promoting fluid production, invigorating Qi and regulating stomach. *Herba Lophatheri* is rich in flavonoids and polysaccharides which can scavenge free radicals in the body and has antibacterial, anticancer, anti-aging and other effects. Raw *Gypsum Fibrosum* and *Radix Ophiopogonis* can regulate the function of macrophages and reticular cells. *Radix Glycyrrhizae* has anti-inflammatory, anti-oxidation and anti-tumor effects.

The prescription is added with *Radix Panacis Quinquefolii*, *Radix Adenophorae*, *Radix Glehniae*, *Fructus Schisandrae Chinensis*, *Folium Mori*, *Rhizoma Phragmitis*, and *Radix Salviae Miltiorrhizae*. *Radix Panacis Quinquefolii* has anti-fatigue, anti-hypoxia, anti-cancer, cardiovascular protection effects and can reduce platelet aggregation, regulate cellular immunity, and protect liver injury. *Radix Adenophorae* and *Radix Glehniae* have antitussive and expectorant effects and can used for the treatment of respiratory diseases. *Radix Glehniae* also has antipyretic, analgesic and immunity enhancing effects. *Fructus Schisandrae Chinensis* has protective effects on central nervous system, liver, immune function and cardiovascular system. In addition, *Fructus Schisandrae Chinensis* can stimulate respiratory system, deepening and accelerating respiration. *Folium Mori* can also be used to treat cough, improve eyesight, quench thirst, reduce blood pressure and regulate lipid metabolism. *Rhizoma Phragmitis* has liver protective, antibacterial, anti-inflammatory and other effects and can be used for bronchitis, acute tonsillitis and common cold.

Indications

The prescription is suitable for patients with fatigue, shortness of breath, dry mouth, thirst, palpitation, hyperhidrosis, anorexia, low heat or non-heat, dry cough with less phlegm, dry tongue with less fluid, and thin pulse or asthenia. *Guidelines for the Diagnosis and Treatment of COVID-19* (Tentative 7th Edition) recommends the prescription for convalescent patients.

Dosage and Administration

Guidelines for the Diagnosis and Treatment of COVID-19 (Tentative 7th Edition) recommends 1 dose per day with 400ml decoction prepared with water by two separate serves with one in the morning and the other in the evening.

Precautions

1. *Radix Panacis Quinquefolii* can cause allergic reactions and aggravate adverse reactions such as arrhythmia and female endocrine disorders.

2. *Fructus Schisandrae Chinensis* can cause gastric acid or stomachache in some patients and is not recommended for long-term application.

3. *Radix Glehniae* can cause allergic dermatitis.

4. Zhuye Shigao Decoction is of cool and moist nature and is restricted for patients with phlegm-dampness or Yang deficiency and fever.

5. *Herba Lophatheri* is of cold nature and patients with spleen and stomach deficiency should not use it.

References

[1] LU J Z, ZHANG Z, ZHAO H, et al. Research on the correspondence between formula and syndrome in Zhuye Shigao Decoction [J] . China Journal of Traditional Chinese Medicine and Pharmacy, 2011, 26 (12): 58-60.

[2] SHU S J. Research progress in pharmacology of American ginseng and its active components [J] . Lishizhen Medicine and Materia Medica Research, 2006, 17 (12): 2603-2604.

[3] CHEN W H. Comparison of modern pharmacological actions of Sargassum from South and North [J] . The Chinese and foreign health abstract, 2008, 5 (4): 251-253.

[4] GUO L Q, ZHANG P, HUANG L L, et al. Research progress on pharmacological action of *Fructus Schisandrae Chinensis* [J] . Acta Chinese Medicine and Pharmacology, 2006, 34 (4): 51-53.

[5] SUN S L. Pharmacological action and clinical application of reed root [J] . Cardiovascular Disease Journal Of integrated traditional Chinese and Western Medicine, 2016, 4 (36): 165.

▌后　记

感谢在本手册出版过程中无私奉献的所有同道!

首先感谢国家卫生健康委员会和国家中医药管理局,连续七版《新型冠状病毒肺炎诊疗方案》的发布,每一版诊疗方案都结合临床实际,与时俱进,为全国迅速有效控制疫情,打赢疫情防控阻击战提供了第一手资料。

感谢辛苦奋战在抗疫一线的所有医务工作者,没有你们舍身忘我的诊疗经验积累,就不会有对疾病的深入认识和科学诊疗方案的面世。在这场没有硝烟却艰险异常的战争中,你们是绝对的"抗疫主力军",是义无反顾的"最美逆行者",也是当之无愧的"最可爱的人"。

感谢人民卫生出版社各位领导和编辑为本手册出版所付出的辛劳和努力,使本手册能够在第一时间得以面世,为抗疫一线医务工作者提供用药参考,为全国各地早日复工、复产、复耕、复学提供坚实基础,这种敬业精神令我们由衷钦佩。

本手册所列药物参照《新型冠状病毒肺炎诊疗方案(试行第七版)》,随着进一步摸索临床诊疗方法和总结临床用药经验,更多药物完成临床试验,更多诊疗手段得以证明,有些药物可能会在后续版本的诊疗方案中被淘汰,有些疗效好的药物会被增补其中,我们将与时俱进,对新冠肺炎药物指导手册进行修订。

　　在以习近平同志为核心的党中央坚强领导下,在全国各级党委和政府的不懈努力下,加之全体医务工作者和科技工作者的辛勤工作,广大人民群众全力以赴、众志成城,一定能够共克时艰,早日迎来抗击疫情阻击战的全面胜利!

Postscript

Thanks to all fellow workers who contribute to the publication of this manual！

Special thanks to the National Health Commission and the State Administration of Traditional Chinese Medicine for the release of seven successive editions of *Guidelines for the Diagnosis and Treatment of COVID-19 (Tentative)*. Every editions are evolved from the past and ongoing clinical practice and trials and contain the most up-to-date knowledge and information pertinent to COVID-19, providing invaluable firsthand information and instructions for the rapid and effective control of the epidemic.

Thanks to all the health care professionals for their self-sacrifice spirit and hard work in fighting against the epidemic. Without your experience in diagnosis and treatment, there would be no in-depth understanding of the disease neither sufficient scientific diagnosis, effective therapeutic approaches and appropriate management strategies. In this life-threatening war, you are absolutely the "main force against the epidemic", "heroes in harm's way" and the "most lovely people". We are truly impressed by their dedication and self-sacrifice spirit.

Thanks to all the leaders and editors of the People's Medical Publishing House for their great efforts that make the publication of this manual possible. Thanks to Prof. Zhiguo Wang for his assistance in the proofreading of this manual. This manual provides some useful reference information on therapeutic drugs and medicines for COVID-19 and the related health problems to the front-line professionals fighting in the anti-epidemic battlefield.

The drugs and medicines described in this manual refer to *Guidelines for the Diagnosis and Treatment of COVID-19* (Tentative 7th Edition). At present, many clinical trials are on the way and the results will soon be released with most up-to-date understanding/ knowledge and technologies/skills for more rapid and accurate diagnosis and more efficient and thorough treatment of COVID-19. We will keep pace with the times and revise the manual timely and accordingly.

We can foresee that under the leadership of President Xi Jinping and the Central Committee of Communist Party of China and with the tireless efforts from our governments at all levels and all medical organizations and health care professionals as well, we will be in no doubt able to overcome all difficulties and harshness around us and conclude the war against COVID-19 with the final win at an early date!

Appendix (Terms of Traditional Chinese Medicine)

Terms	Annotation	Appearance
Bitter/ Pungent	the five tastes of medicinals, pungency, sweetness, sourness, bitterness, and saltiness, representing the basic actions of the medicinals	Lianhua Qingwen Capsule (Granules) ; Prescription for Syndrome of Cold-dampness Stagnation in Lung; Prescription for Syndrome of Accumulation of Dampness-Heat in Lung; Prescription for Syndrome of Epidemic Pathogen Blocking Lung; Prescription for Syndrome of Dual Blaze of Qi Nutrient Aspects
Blood-tonifying	a therapeutic method to treat blood deficiency by using blood-tonifying medicinals, the same as to nourish or restore blood	Huoxiang Zhengqi Capsule (Pill, Water, Oral Liquid) ; Shuanghuanglian Oral Liquid (Powder Injection) ; Gelanxiang Oral Liquid
Cold-dampness	a combined pathogen of cold and dampness	Prescription for Syndrome of Cold-dampness Stagnation in Lung; Prescription for Syndrome of Cold-Dampness Obstructing Lung

Continue

Terms	Annotation	Appearance
Dampness	dampness as a pathogenic factor characterized by its impediment to Qi movement and its turbidity, heaviness, stickiness and downward flowing properties, also called pathogenic dampness	Qingfei Huatan Pill; Huatan Juhong Oral Liquid; Jinzhen Oral Liquid; Jinhua Qinggan Granules; Huoxiang Zhengqi Capsule (Pill, Water, Oral Liquid) ; Qingfei Paidu Decoction; Prescription for Syndrome of Cold-dampness Stagnation in Lung; Prescription for Syndrome of Accumulation of Dampness-Heat in Lung; Prescription for Syndrome of Stagnation of Dampness Toxin in Lung; Prescription for Syndrome of Cold-Dampness Obstructing Lung; Prescription for Syndrome of Dual Blaze of Qi Nutrient Aspects; Prescription for Syndrome of Qi Deficiency of Lung and Spleen; Prescription for Syndrome of Dual Deficiency of Qi and Yin
Damp-ness-Heat	a combined pathogen of dampness and heat	Prescription for Syndrome of Accumulation of Dampness-Heat in Lung
Dampness Toxin	noxious pathogenic factor formed by stagnation of dampness, which may cause hematochezia when it occurs in the intestine, or ulcer of the shank when in the muscles and skin of the lower limbs	Prescription for Syndrome of Stagnation of Dampness Toxin in Lung

Continue

Terms	Annotation	Appearance
Fire	a pathogenic factor that causes heat pattern/ syndrome, also called pathogenic heat	Jinzhen Oral Liquid; Lianhua Qingwen Capsule (Granules) ; Shuanghuanglian Oral Liquid (Powder Injection) ; Qingfei Paidu Decoction; Prescription for Syndrome of Internal Block and External Collapse; Prescription for Syndrome of Qi Deficiency of Lung and Spleen
Harmonize the stomach	therapeutic method to treat dysfunction of the stomach	Jinzhen Oral Liquid; Prescription for Syndrome of Qi Deficiency of Lung and Spleen
Heat	heat as a pathogenic factor that causes heat pattern/syndrome, also called pathogenic heat	Qingfei Huatan Pill; Qutanling Oral Liquid; Huatan Juhong Oral Liquid; Jinzhen Oral Liquid; Jinhua Qinggan Granules; Lianhua Qingwen Capsule (Granules) ; Shufeng Jiedu Capsule (Granules) ; Fangfeng Tongsheng Pill (Granules) ; Shuanghuanglian Oral Liquid (Powder Injection) ; Gelanxiang Oral Liquid; Xingnaojing Injection; Xuebijing Injection; Reduning Injection; Shenfu Injection; Shenmai Injection; Qingfei Paidu Decoction; Prescription for Syndrome of Cold-dampness Stagnation in Lung; Prescription for Syndrome of Accumulation of Dampness-Heat in Lung; Prescription for Syndrome of Cold-Dampness Obstructing Lung; Prescription for Syndrome of Internal Block and External

Continue

Terms	Annotation	Appearance
Heat		Collapse; Prescription for Syndrome of Qi Deficiency of Lung and Spleen; Prescription for Syndrome of Dual Deficiency of Qi and Yin
Lung meridian	one of the regular twelve meridians which begins internally in the middle energizer, descends to connect with the large intestine, then ascends to the lung and throat, courses laterally and exits superficially at zhongfu (LU1) , and then descends along the lateral side of the arm and forearm, terminates at shaoshang (LU11) , with 11 acupuncture points on either side	Jinhua Qinggan Granules
Middle energizer	the upper abdominal cavity, i. e. , the portion between the diaphragm and the umbilicus housing the spleen, stomach, liver and gallbladder, also known as middle burner	Prescription for Syndrome of Cold-dampness Stagnation in Lung

Continue

Terms	Annotation	Appearance
Qi	In the field of medicine, Qi refers both to the refined nutritive substance that flows within the human body as well as to its functional activities	Qingfei Huatan Pill; Huatan Juhong Oral Liquid; Jinzhen Oral Liquid; Huoxiang Zhengqi Capsule (Pill, Water, Oral Liquid) ; Fangfeng Tongsheng Pill; Shuanghuanglian Oral Liquid (Powder Injection) ; Gelanxiang Oral Liquid; Shengmai Injection; Shenfu Injection; Shenmai Injection; Qingfei Paidu Decoction; Prescription for Syndrome of Cold-dampness Stagnation in Lung; Prescription for Syndrome of Cold-Dampness Obstructing Lung; Prescription for Syndrome of Dual Blaze of Qi Nutrient Aspects; Prescription for Syndrome of Internal Block and External Collapse; Prescription for Syndrome of Qi Deficiency of Lung and Spleen; Prescription for Syndrome of Dual Deficiency of Qi and Yin
Removing stagnation	promote digestion and remove food stagnation	Huoxiang Zhengqi Capsule (Pill, Water, Oral Liquid)
Repelling foulness	a therapeutic method of using aromatic medicinals to treat diseases caused by pathogenic foul turbidity	Huoxiang Zhengqi Capsule (Pill, Water, Oral Liquid)

Continue

Terms	Annotation	Appearance
Restore Yang	a therapeutic method of using a large dose of warm or hot-natured medicinals to prevent the patient from collapsing	Shenfu Injection
Stomach cold	a pathological change either due to deficiency of stomach Yang or caused by direct attack of pathogenic cold, the former being deficiency-cold of the stomach, and the latter, excess-cold in the stomach	Prescription for Syndrome of Dual Blaze of Qi Nutrient Aspects
Syndrome of dual blaze of Qi nutrient aspects	a pattern/syndrome characterized by simultaneous existence of syndromes of Qi and nutrient aspects, manifested by high fever, thirst, mental irritability, delirium and barely visible skin eruption	Prescription for Syndrome of Dual Blaze of Qi Nutrient Aspects

Continue

Terms	Annotation	Appearance
Syndrome of dual deficiency of Qi and Yin	a pattern/syndrome marked by listlessness, lack of strength, shortness of breath, reluctance to speak, dry throat and mouth, vexing thirst, flushed cheeks in the afternoon, short voidings of small amount of urine, constipation, emaciation, scanty dry tongue coating and vacuous pulse	Prescription for Syndrome of Dual Deficiency of Qi and Yin
Syndrome of internal block and external collapse	a pattern/syndrome in which excess pathogens are trapped in the interior (as manifested by fever, cough and dyspnea, or by abdominal pain with tenesmus, or by constipation and urinary block, or by colicky pain in the chest, epigastrium and abdomen) while the healthy Qi collapses (as manifested by pallor, reversal cold of limbs, cold dripping sweats, feeble breathing and scarcely perceptible pulse)	Prescription for Syndrome of Internal Block and External Collapse

Continue

Terms	Annotation	Appearance
Unsur-faced fever	a persistent fever in which heat is not easily felt on the body surface and can be felt only by prolonged palpation, a sign of dampness-heat	Prescription for Syndrome of Cold-Dampness Obstructing Lung
Upper energizer	the chest cavity, i. e. , the portion above the dia-phragm housing the heart and lung, also known as upper burner	Lianhua Qingwen Capsule (Gra-nules)
Warm disease	a general term for acute externally transmit-ted diseases caused by warm pathogens, with fever as the chief mani-festation, also known as warm pathogen disease	Shuanghuanglian Oral Liquid (Pow-der Injection) ; Xuebijing Injec-tion; Prescription for Syndrome of Internal Block and External Collapse
Wind	wind as a pathogenic fac-tor characterized by its rapid movement, swift changes, and ascending and opening actions, also called pathogenic wind	Qingfei Huatan Pill; Shufeng Jiedu Capsule (Granules)
Wind-heat	a combined pathogen of external wind and heat	Huatan Juhong Oral Liquid; Jinhua Qinggan Granules; Shufeng Jiedu Cap-sule (Granules) ; Shuanghuanglian Oral Liquid (Powder Injection) ; Gelanxiang Oral Liquid; Reduning Injection; Qing-fei Paidu Decoction

Continue

Terms	Annotation	Appearance
Wind-cold	a combined pathogen of external wind and cold	Qingfei Huatan Pill; Jinzhen Oral Liquid; Huoxiang Zhengqi Capsule (Pill, Water, Oral Liquid) ; Lianhua Qingwen Capsule (Granules) ; Fangfeng Tongsheng Pill (Granules) ; Shuanghuanglian Oral Liquid (Powder Injection) ; Qingfei Paidu Decoction
Yin	In Chinese philosophy, the feminine, latent and passive principle (characterized by dark, cold, wetness, passivity, disintegration, etc.) of the two opposing cosmic forces into which creative energy divides and whose fusion in physical matter brings the phenomenal world into being	Huoxiang Zhengqi Capsule (Pill, Water, Oral Liquid) ; Fangfeng Tongsheng Pill (Granules) ; Shuanghuanglian Oral Liquid (Powder Injection) ; Gelanxiang Oral Liquid; Shengmai Injection; Shenfu Injection; Shenmai Injection; Qingfei Paidu Decoction; Prescription for Syndrome of Cold-Dampness Obstructing Lung; Prescription for Syndrome of Epidemic Pathogen Blocking Lung; Prescription for Syndrome of Dual Blaze of Qi Nutrient Aspects; Prescription for Syndrome of Internal Block and External Collapse; Prescription for Syndrome of Dual Deficiency of Qi and Yin
Yang	In Chinese philosophy, the masculine, active and positive principle (characterized by light, warmth, dryness, activity, etc.) of the two opposing cosmic forces into which creative energy divides and whose fusion in physical matter brings the phenomenal world into being	Huoxiang Zhengqi Capsule (Pill, Water, Oral Liquid) ; Fangfeng Tongsheng Pill (Granules) ; Shuanghuanglian Oral Liquid (Powder Injection) ; Gelanxiang Oral Liquid; Shenfu Injection; Qingfei Paidu Decoction; Prescription for Syndrome of Internal Block and External Collapse; Prescription for Syndrome of Qi Deficiency of Lung and Spleen; Prescription for Syndrome of Dual Deficiency of Qi and Yin

08柱